RC
961.5
.B43

N. TECH. UNIV. LI
343
ack N.
ases : responses

Tropical Diseases
Responses of
Pharmaceutical Companies

Jack N. Behrman

American Enterprise Institute for Public Policy Research
Washington and London

Tennessee Tech. Library
Cookeville, Tenn.

303382

Jack N. Behrman is Luther Hodges Distinguished Professor of Business Administration at the University of North Carolina at Chapel Hill.

Library of Congress Cataloging in Publication Data

Behrman, Jack N
    Tropical diseases.

    (AEI studies; 288)
    1. Tropical medicine—Social aspects.   2. Underdeveloped areas—Pharmaceutical policy.   3. Pharmaceutical research—Tropics.   4. Underdeveloped areas–Medical policy.   5. Schistosomiasis—Brazil.   I. Title.   II. Series: American Enterprise Institute for Public Policy Research. AEI studies; 288.
    RC961.5.B43   362.1'0913   80–20164
    ISBN 0–8447–3393–8

AEI Studies 288

© 1980 by the American Enterprise Institute for Public Policy Research, Washington and London. All rights reserved. No part of this publication may be used or reproduced in any manner whatsoever without permission in writing from the American Enterprise Institute except in the case of brief quotations embodied in news articles, critical articles, or reviews.

The views expressed in the publications of the American Enterprise Institute are those of the authors and do not necessarily reflect the views of the staff, advisory panels, officers, or trustees of AEI.

"American Enterprise Institute" and ⬭ are registered service marks of the American Enterprise Institute for Public Policy Research.

Printed in the United States of America

Contents

Preface

In recent years both the World Health Organization (WHO) and some members of the U.S. Congress have asked whether American and European pharmaceutical companies are doing as much as they might to eradicate tropical disease in the developing nations. Currently, malaria, schistosomiasis, and other tropical diseases are responsible for thousands of deaths and untold cases of illness in Asia, Africa, and Latin America each year. The secondary effects of these diseases include reduced economic productivity, lowered physical vitality, and mental lethargy.

This book examines what the pharmaceutical companies have done in the past to combat the six most prevalent tropical diseases and what they are doing today, both within their own laboratories and in conjunction with health agencies in developing countries. In addition, the book includes a case study of a major Brazilian program to control schistosomiasis.

The Brazilian program was examined at firsthand by the author, and the case study is based on interviews with officials of the Brazilian government, observation of program activities in the field, and a review of documents provided by Brazilian officials. Other chapters are based primarily on personal interviews of drug company officials, although a number of published papers also proved helpful. Company officials were assured during the interviews that their statements would not be attributed if they felt that otherwise the review and approval process within their companies would seriously delay the study and, possibly, prevent publication. To make certain that the information in the paper was accurate, portions of the report on the activities of particular companies were read by company officials, but presentation of the interview results remains the sole responsibility of the author.

Acknowledgment and thanks are herewith extended not only to the pharmaceutical companies and their representatives who consented to be interviewed, but also to the Pharmaceutical Manufacturers Association and the International Federation of Pharmaceutical

Manufacturers Association who provided useful information. The author also expresses his appreciation to the Fund for Multinational Management Education of New York City, which sponsored and administered the research project.

1

Tropical Diseases in Developing Countries: An International Perspective

The primary requisites for good health—often lacking in tropical countries—are, of course, good nutrition, potable water, sanitation, and methods for health care and maintenance. In addition, direct attacks on the causes and cures of diseases are required. Specific health care needs vary among the developing countries because of differences in climate, education, and social and economic development. Even where needs are similar, the reception and use of modern pharmaceuticals (drugs) vary considerably, reflecting contributions of governments to health care, campaigns against specific diseases, and cultural differences among countries. Some areas still rely on traditional medicine, rather than modern (scientific) drugs. Even where such ethical drugs are available, education as to their appropriate use and the need to consult physicians varies among countries, as does the availability of local medical help.

The use of drugs in developing countries ranges widely with the degree to which people are accustomed to self-medication, with the prescribing practices of doctors, and with the availability of public health services (especially in rural areas) and of hospitals. Also, countries differ in their reliance on generic drugs or proprietary drugs. Countries differ in the degree that drugs are in constant supply (whether from local production or imports) and in the extent to which they are available to the public directly through retail outlets or only through physicians. And differences exist in the degree to which major campaigns are oriented through public health services.

The pharmaceutical companies rarely participate in large preventive campaigns or general health care programs. Rather, they come in at a late stage in health programs. Although some of them have also participated in programs to control the disease carriers or

1

sources, their main activity is in remedies after a disease has been contracted.

The pharmaceutical industry is predominately in the business of supplying drugs to health units or physicians. But the process of doing so requires the invention, production, quality control, and monitoring of pharmaceutical products and the distribution of these products to physicians, hospitals, pharmacies, and public health services. The pharmaceutical companies respond to market pulls for the drugs—both in production and in research on particular diseases. In developing countries, funds for purchases of drugs come mostly from governmental budgets. The funds for health care remain relatively low, however, averaging between 1 and 2 percent of GNP, and only 15 to 30 percent of these funds may be spent on drugs. Moreover, the governments' budgets are frequently spent on eradication of single diseases, rather than on the treatment of individuals, which would include a wide spectrum of illnesses. This approach is taken partly because public health services are provided inadequate funds to take care of the wide range of diseases they would like to control. Therefore, many patients turn to, or are directed to, the private sector, where a larger variety of drugs is available.

Since the pharmaceutical companies respond to market demands, and since many governments do not adequately fund programs for removing widespread diseases, a gap has developed between the need to remove some specific diseases and the efforts by the pharmaceutical research community. When this gap is considered in the context of the quite adequate research efforts undertaken by the pharmaceutical industry to meet diseases and health care problems of the types found in advanced countries, invidious comparisons are sometimes made, despite the fact that many diseases in Europe and North America are also common in developing countries. Yet, the work on problems common to both areas does require additional effort to meet needs of developing countries. The stability of medicaments for developing countries must be adapted to the climate and conditions of storage; they must be safe and simple to use as they are often administered by paramedical personnel. Many infectious diseases prevalent in developed countries are also significant in warm climates—such as those due to viruses (measles, hepatitis) or bacteria (pneumonia, otitis, tuberculosis, venereal diseases). Other problems such as hereditary blood diseases, hypertension, and contraception are of major importance in less-developed countries (LDCs). Since markets in the advanced countries are adequate to induce research on these, the developing countries benefit— whether or not they give these diseases the highest priority—and

2

their needs are being adequately met by current efforts of the pharmaceutical companies.

But a significant gap exists between needs and capabilities in dealing with many diseases indigenous to tropical countries. Among these, the more important are malaria, schistosomiasis, and filariasis. Less pervasive are trypanosomiasis, leishmaniasis, and leprosy. Each of the three major diseases affects more than 200 million people; they cause continued absence from work and frequently permanent incapacitation or death.[1] Present means to combat these diseases are inadequate, because drugs are not available or cannot be delivered into rural communities. The three minor diseases are also not yet eradicable. Some of these diseases have multiple sources, complicating the processes of drug development and application.

Malaria

Malaria, which is a fever spread by mosquitoes, causes more than a million deaths a year, mostly in tropical Africa. Despite extensive efforts to eradicate it in several areas, it is still widespread; eradication is made difficult by a variety of operational, financial, and technical obstacles. The operational obstacles are lack of administrative personnel, organizational deficiencies, and the paucity of trained technicians. The financial difficulties reflect insufficient budget allocations in particular countries or a lack of resources to allocate for social purposes. The technical difficulties stem from the fact that some of the mosquitoes modify their behavior to reduce contact with insecticides spread on the walls and develop resistance to the insecticides, which are also widely used in agriculture. Furthermore, some of the parasites carrying the disease also develop resistance to drugs. Population shifts and other factors make these obstacles more difficult to overcome.

Schistosomiasis

Schistosomiasis (snail fever, or bilharzia) is a slow-developing infection of the liver and blood stream of a person, which takes several years to show symptoms. It exists in seventy-one countries and is spreading because of migration and increased contacts among people

---

[1] The data on the six diseases discussed in this and succeeding sections are taken from World Health Organization, *Special Programme for Research and Training in Tropical Diseases* (Geneva: Vols. I and II. Docs. TDR/PK/76.1 (1976) and TDR/WK/76.3 (1976).

and, above all, because of irrigation programs which permit the spread of snails that are hosts to the parasites.

The parasites are three different types of blood flukes or flat worms, barely visible to the eye. Three different forms of the disease result, found in three different areas of the world; their effects on the human hosts are different, though the disease is essentially the same. In the process of infection, the human is entered by worms that have gestated in an intermediate snail host, which lives in a warm water environment used also by humans. When in humans, male and female adult worms combine in nearly continuous copulation for a lifetime of four to fourteen years, producing many thousands of eggs each day in the tissues. Some of the eggs escape in human feces, frequently excreted into water used in the community. Once in the water, the eggs burst, releasing a larva with a lifespan of about twenty-four hours, which seeks a suitable fresh water snail as its host. Once in the snail, the larvae multiply to form thousands of cercaria, or baby worms, which leave the snail in search of humans. When anyone steps into the water or reaches in, the small worm bores through the skin, settling in the blood vessels of various internal organs, and begins the cycle again.

The disease causes lesions and sometimes dysentery, hypertension, or pulmonary or cardiac complications, as well as urinary infection and various renal complications. More technically, schistosomiasis produces liver dysfunction that can lead to gastric hemorrhage and consequently acute anemia, hypoproteinemia ascites, hyperspleenism, and infantilism. The lungs may also be affected, leading to corpulmonale, followed by cardiac failure, or cyanosis; the intestines can become involved, and, finally, some neurological disorder may occur. The severe form of the disease begins to appear only after the sixth year of age despite the fact that infection usually is contracted the first years of life, as children play around and in the water of the village. The most serious form is developed only between the nineteenth and twentieth years and is highly correlated with numbers of worms in the body and the number of eggs produced by them, passing through in the feces. Many symptoms are evident to the patient only after some years, as pain or debility intensifies.

Schistosomiasis is normally a rural disease, associated with poor sanitation facilities. It also strikes those engaged in agricultural or fishing activities that place them near fresh water. Control of schistosomiasis depends on—(1) keeping human excreta from getting into the water; (2) reducing the population of snails; (3) reducing human contact with infected water through better sanitation and water supply; and (4) reducing the number of persons spreading the disease, through treatment of those infected.

Filariasis

Filariasis is also caused by parasitic worms and is manifested in several forms, including onchocerciasis, guinea worm infection, and elephantiasis. All forms cause extreme pain and impairment of general health, including blindness. Elephantiasis is the swelling and deformation of the extremities and afflicts over 200 million people; onchocerciasis is the most severe form of the disease, involving some 30 million; guinea worm, affecting the face and eyes (a subcutaneous form that can reach several feet), affects some 10 million persons. A minor form (loiasis) invokes subcutaneous and perarticular swelling, and afflicts some 1 million persons. Only two drugs are of use in these diseases, both introduced over thirty years ago, with no relevant discovery since then in this field. Present treatment of the disease requires a two-to-seven-week course of medication.

The adult worms take between three and fifteen months to mature, according to their species, and survive up to fifteen years in a human host, where they are deposited by the bite of an insect. Each small worm injected does not multiply, as in schistosomiasis, but grows up as one worm in the human. A buildup of the disease in an individual, therefore, requires repeated exposure to infection. The adult worm produces larvae, which settle in various parts of the body of the host causing the symptoms of the disease and the damage to various tissues, including the eyes (producing "river blindness"). The cycle is continued when the carrier insect (vector) ingests the larvae by biting the human hosts in the area of the infection; the larvae develop as worms in the insect and are ready to be injected into a human host when the insect feeds again.

Trypanosomiasis, Leishmaniasis, and Leprosy

Trypanosomiasis is found in Africa and South America in different forms. African sleeping sickness extends from lower West Africa across the tropical belt into northern South Africa. Large-scale control measures have reduced the incidence of the disease to low endemic levels, but it flares up when control measures are discontinued. At least 35 million people are exposed to the disease and 10,000 new cases are known to occur every year. An estimated 10 million people exposed to the disease are examined yearly by mobile medical teams (composed of national and international personnel) at a cost of some

5

$5 million (U.S.). Much larger amounts, probably over ten times more, are spent by public and private sources to control the tsetse fly, which is the carrier of the disease. These large amounts are spent in part to protect animals against the disease.

When the infected flies bite humans (or animals) they inject the parasites under the skin, and the parasites flow into the bloodstream. In humans, the results are fever, headaches, and pains in the joints; later on, there is damage to the central nervous system, leading to psychosis, somnolence, and coma. Early diagnosis of the disease is difficult, because the symptoms are similar to flu or malaria. Later diagnosis requires sophisticated tests not always available in the field. The South American trypanosomiasis (Chagas' disease) has a much higher incidence than the African form. It usually has a better prognosis than the sleeping sickness, although the mortality in small children or in adults after a ten-to-twenty-year duration might be higher than is usually thought.

Leishmaniasis is the collective name for a variety of infections caused by parasites that affect several million people. The results of infestation may be simply a sore, or spreading sores, or disfiguring lesions and ulcerated tissues, or they may be of the biserral type known as kala-aza, which is usually fatal when not treated. Leishmaniasis exists in all continents save Australia and Antarctica—though it is absent from most of Southeast Asia, the United States, and large areas of tropical Africa. It is transmitted by the bite of sandflies, which also feed on domestic and forest animals. Although few statistics are available on the prevalence of the disease, biserral leishmaniasis occurred in some 77,000 newly infected patients on the Indian subcontinent in the 1950s. Only the spraying of DDT during an antimalarial campaign brought it under control, by reducing the sandfly population; but when this insecticide was discontinued, the disease returned.

Leprosy also remains a problem in many developing countries, where between 11 and 12 million cases exist, concentrated principally in tropical countries. The disease causes skin lesions and scaling and is serious enough to develop deformities in about one-third of the cases. It is feared in many communities though its frequency of transmittal by humans is no greater than some other diseases; as a consequence, lepers are often segregated into colonies.

These diseases are the subject of continuing research and developing programs by several pharmaceutical companies, but not all of the major companies are so engaged, and none has a complete program in all diseases. The World Health Organization (WHO) has, however, selected these six diseases for a special program of control or eradication.

The Special Program of the World Health Organization

In 1976, WHO adopted a "Special Programme for Research and Training in Tropical Diseases." The objective was not only to draw attention to the impact of the six diseases just discussed but also to help prioritize them. It placed malaria first, followed by schistosomiasis, trypanosomiasis, filariasis, leprosy, and leishmaniasis. The program seeks "to develop and apply new diagnostic methods, chemotherapeutic agents and vaccines especially suited to prevent and treat the diseases of the tropics in the countries affected by them," and "to strengthen research in the countries affected by the diseases by training of scientists and technicians in the relevant disciplines."[2] These two goals are seen as complementary and requiring simultaneous efforts. The training of scientists and development of institutes in developing countries are required in order to transfer technology from the advanced countries successfully. The program is also concerned with systems for delivery of medications and the creation of an appropriate local (social and cultural) environment in which to administer the drugs and control other features contributing to the diseases.

WHO has set up separate research task forces for each of the six diseases; these groups collaborate with existing laboratories—university, company, independent, or governmental—in both developing and advanced countries. Laboratories in developing countries receive financial and technical assistance to help create national centers of research and research training. Support is given for international multidisciplinary research centers in regions where the diseases are endemic and where research resources are of the type necessary to undertake specific projects. Research training will be provided at these interdisciplinary centers, supported mainly by the host nations.

The director general of WHO, in a speech presenting his *Annual Report* for 1976, called for more and better public health training in LDCs:

> One of the most serious obstacles to country health programming is the lack of personnel trained to apply the process. It is lamentable that most schools of public health provide training that does little or nothing to motivate and

---

[2] Ibid.

equip future health executives to strengthen the process of health development in their countries and fuse it with other developmental efforts for the satisfaction of basic human needs. The support of learning for this purpose has thus become a major challenge for WHO.[3]

In a prior speech, he had emphasized that eradication programs were dependent also on the level of economic development in the countries concerned:

> In the malaria and smallpox eradication programs we can see instances of broad campaigns where WHO has learned from its mistakes and has continued to learn from them. The main lesson learned is that, in the fight against disease, too much emphasis must not be placed on health technologies alone. What we can achieve in this field depends directly on the level of economic development in the countries concerned.[4]

The malaria programs in many countries were seen by the task forces as inadequately linked to the infrastructure of local health services or the prior creation of adequate community services to reduce exposure to the disease. As a consequence of its experiences in malaria, WHO's Special Program emphasizes the development of inexpensive but necessary tools and techniques to control diseases—better diagnosis, improved therapies, and control of vectors (parasite carriers)—requiring minimum skill levels and integrated into local public health services. The program also seeks to strengthen biomedical research in tropical countries directed at developing, specifying, and testing the necessary tools and techniques of control. These require manpower development and the strengthening of research, primarily in the tropical countries but also in advanced-country laboratories. WHO will coordinate each of the programs on the six diseases, but scientific and technical advisory committees, including industry representatives, will help oversee them. In particular, WHO plans to provide facilities for the clinical-pharmacological evaluation of new drugs, minimizing the delay between preclinical experimentation and clinical use. WHO believes that it must work with and encourage the pharmaceutical industry to reverse a declining interest in R & D on tropical diseases. It hopes, by the Special Program, to assure the industry that WHO has a continuing interest in antiparasitic drugs.[5]

---

[3] Address by Dr. H. Mahler, 30th World Health Assembly, Press Release WHA/3, May 3, 1977, p. 3.
[4] *WHO Features*, no. 36, April 1976, p. 2.
[5] WHO *Special Programme on Research*, TDR/PK/76.1.

For each of the six diseases, WHO has established a review panel composed of researchers from various laboratories, including those of pharmaceutical companies, as well as government and public health officials. The task of the panels has been to get the existing information on the diseases, describe present control measures, suggest a role for WHO in the promotion of research, and outline a program for each disease.

WHO wishes to stimulate greater attention to disease control by the host countries—which, in WHO's view, can bear 80 to 90 percent of the cost of control programs through contributions of local manpower and resources. If these local funds were forthcoming they would provide an attractive market for the pharmaceutical companies, stimulating their interest in developing appropriate medications. WHO has recognized that underutilization of existing drugs has deterred new efforts at drug development by private industry, and that a remedy for this situation begins with an increase in funding by the countries for expansion of disease control.[6]

---

[6] M. Marois, ed., *Development of Chemotherapeutic Agents for Parasitic Diseases*, Proceedings of WHO/Pharmaceutical Industry Conference, Versailles, June 1974 (Paris: l'Institute de la Vie, 1974).

2

Pharmaceutical Company Activities

Several pharmaceutical companies are involved in developing drugs for the six parasitic diseases. Some of the larger companies dedicate fairly substantial efforts to R & D on tropical diseases: for example, Lepetit in Italy; Bayer, Hoechst and Merck (Darmstadt) in Germany; Wellcome, Beecham, and S. Ross in Britain; Janssen in Belgium; Roche and Ciba-Geigy in Switzerland; Rhône-Poulenc in France; plus Sterling-Winthrop, Merck, Pfizer, and Warner-Lambert/Parke-Davis in the United States. Others are peripherally or indirectly involved; and, of course, research is being undertaken also by private and governmental institutes or laboratories.

Efforts are also being made by companies in the development and distribution of drugs for a variety of other diseases and health conditions; in the support of delivery systems in both the private and the public sectors; and in cooperative projects in both research and training of professional health personnel. The cooperative projects are discussed in chapter 3; the direct activities are described here.

Not all companies are involved in each activity. Indeed, not only do companies assume different roles but each tends to specialize in particular areas of pharmacology or types of disease. Some are involved in both chemotherapy and immunology, whereas others give little attention to the development of vaccines. Almost all provide technical assistance and manpower training to LDCs. The various company activities and experiences are described to illustrate their scope, nature, and location. Since no effort is made to detail all that is being done, the record here is not complete for all companies.

To date the following drugs have been made available or are being tested for treatment of the six tropical diseases:

- *Malaria:* after quinine, acranil derivatives and chloroquine, new compounds have been developed: acedapsone, amodiaquine, amopyroquine, proguanil, primaquine, chlorproguanil, cycloguanil pamoate, pyrimethamine, sulfalene, sulfonamide + pyrimethamine combination, and mefloquine.

- *Schistosomiasis:* after the old antimony derivatives: hycanthone, niridazole, metrifonate, lucanthone hydrochloride, and oxamniquine.
- *Filariasis:* after suramine and diethylcarbamazine, mebendazole and metrifonate may prove useful.
- *Trypanosomiasis:* melarsonyl, melarsoprol, pentamidine isothionate; and nifurtimox; and benznidazol for Chagas' disease.
- *Leprosy:* after solfones, clofazimine, thiambutosine, acedapsone, rifampicin, and various long-acting sulfonamides.
- *Leishmaniasis:* hydroxystilbamadine isothionate, amphotericin B and pentavalent antimony derivatives.

As early as 1962, a study by the Division of Medical Services of the United States National Academy of Sciences/National Research Council declared that only schistosomiasis remained uncontrollable among the six diseases. Leprosy was theoretically controllable by chemotherapy; leishmaniasis and Chagas' disease would still have to be controlled through attacks on the vectors; whereas malaria, trypanosomiasis, and filariasis were more or less controllable through vectors as well as chemotherapy. Among the "six diseases," schistosomiasis was the least effectively controllable,[7] but since 1962 the epidemiological situation for the six diseases has deteriorated, especially for malaria and trypanosomiasis, leaving more persons afflicted and the diseases under less control.

Many of the companies are currently screening chemical compounds for possible use in some or all of the six tropical diseases. This screening is done on an ad hoc basis—that is, a compound is screened only for a particular disease if it appears to be potentially useful. Compounds are not screened for all six diseases on a continuing basis. For example, drugs being developed for tuberculosis will be tested against leprosy, and those for schistosomiasis will be tested against other parasitic diseases, such as leishmaniasis and Chagas' disease. To bring its screening processes closer to the disease location, one company has standing screening agreements covering Chagas' disease, schistosomiasis, and trypanosomiasis, with faculties

---

[7] National Academy of Sciences/National Research Council, *Tropical Health: A Report on a Study of Needs and Resources* (Washington, D.C.: National Academy of Sciences, 1962), pp. 132–33.

in Brazil, Upper Volta, and Thailand; and other companies with university laboratories in Buenos Aires, San Salvador, and elsewhere.

Pfizer, Smith Kline & French, Hoechst, Wellcome, Bayer, and other companies working in veterinary medicine in the areas of parasitology and anthelminthics (worms of various species) have potential spinoffs of these compounds for human use—for trypanosomiasis, for example. Praziquantel from Merck and Bayer has been successful in veterinary medicine and is now being tested for schistosomiasis. This spinoff makes research in the area of the given disease attractive, since the potential drug has a larger market in both animal and human users. One serious complication of the screening of drugs for parasitic diseases is that one drug may work only for a specific form of a disease, while another drug has to be developed for another form of the same disease. For example, some drugs work for *Schistosoma haematobium*, as found in Egypt, but not on *Schistosoma mansoni*. Some drugs are more active in forms of *S. mansoni* found in Brazil than in the African form of the same disease. Each such limitation narrows the market and diminishes research interest.

The following section focuses on the activities of the companies in the six special diseases, on their research on vaccines for immunology, and on their efforts to cure other diseases in developing countries.

Activities in the Six Diseases

Companies differ in their attention to the several diseases but have similar criteria as to nature of research projects to be supported. They simply apply or interpret the criteria differently. Some pharmaceutical companies have decided not to pursue drug development in the six tropical diseases at all; others have unsuccessfully tried for years to develop scientific compounds, as might be the case in any field of medical research.

Drug Development. The following is a brief account of the scope and nature of R & D of several companies on the six diseases.

Pfizer's major work has been in schistosomiasis (see chapter 4). It has done much less on filariasis, malaria, leprosy, or leishmaniasis. It did undertake a project in filariasis some years ago, but concluded that the multiple disease forms involved (several different worms produce the disease, with different life cycles and in different hosts) made it highly unlikely that a single drug would be useful; this, of course, would substantially raise the cost of drug development. In addition, the geographic distribution of the disease makes it difficult to apply treatment effectively.

Parke-Davis began its work in parasitology in 1935, concentrating on the chemotherapy of malaria. This work has broadened to include filariasis, schistosomiasis, intestinal helminthiases (worms), tuberculosis, and leprosy during the period after World War II. In the decade 1960–1969, Parke-Davis invested approximately $16 million in antiparasitic research. During that time, the effort devoted to parasite chemotherapy ranged between 6 and 13 percent of its total annual research. Out of this work, the company developed and marketed seven different drugs for malaria, one for leishmaniasis, and two for leprosy, but it was not successful in developing any for filariasis, trypanosomiasis, or schistosomiasis. It continues, however, to work on schistosomiasis under a grant from the Edna Clark Foundation and on malaria under a contract from the Walter Reed Army Institute of Research (WRAIR).

Janssen (Johnson & Johnson's affiliate in Belgium) has had good results from compounds potentially useful in filariasis and onchocerciasis (a form of filariasis), but a wide range of tests will be necessary before the company can be certain of success. The laboratory is also working on schistosomiasis, applying the drugs to the schistosomiasis found in rats (*S. rodeni*), since rodents (along with dogs) are natural hosts. The company is doing nothing in malaria or leprosy, but has a limited program in leishmaniasis and trypanosomiasis. Two strains of trypanosomiasis are being tested in rodents.

Hoffman-LaRoche has been in tropical disease research since 1953, and is working on five of the six special diseases (not leprosy). Its projects are exceedingly long term, requiring budget allocations for at least fifteen years on each project, though the lab expects to achieve something within ten years—otherwise, in their view, they should not have started any given project. But one project required thirteen years of screening before a useful result was found, and five more years before Phase I clinical trials could be begun with a very few patients. It has two compounds in development in these diseases after fifteen years of effort.

Roche's total research program is divided into three parts, one of which is chemotherapy. Within chemotherapy, there are three major divisions: bacteriology and virology, cancer, and tropical diseases (parasitology and mycology). Tropical disease research absorbs at least one-third of the budget for chemotherapy research, which amounts to 10 percent of the total research budget of the research

13

unit in Basel. The work in the other divisions of the lab is important for tropical diseases, since some basic derivatives of natural antibiotics (such as 2-nitroi-midazoles) have led to a drug for Chagas' disease, the second on the market. Roche's efforts on Chagas' disease show the problems in the development of drugs for the six diseases. In 1959 one of the researchers in the Roche lab read a publication on a new antibiotic, which indicated possible application to one of the forms of trypanosomiasis. By 1964, after five years of screening on Chagas' disease, a newly synthesized compound was found to be very promising by the team in Basel and others working in universities of Brazil. During preclinical research work, neurotoxicity in dogs was observed. However, this toxicity of nitroimidazol derivatives proved to be specific to dogs alone, since the compound was proved safe when tested in other animals. By 1971, clinical tests were begun in several areas, mainly in Latin America, where the disease is endemic. These trials took seven years because of the necessity to follow-up the patients during a two-to-five-year period, including parasitology and immunology. As with filariasis, leishmaniasis, and trypanosomiasis, the natural history of Chagas' disease is not known. The drug was introduced only in 1978, and research work on activity, pharmacokinetics, metabolism, and tolerance still continues. Chagas' disease has been given a top priority in the company because there were no adequate drugs available. Once the company has succeeded for Chagas' disease, priority will shift the resources to African trypanosomiasis.

Roche's research in malaria has led to the development of Fansidar, which is active in the treatment and in the once-a-week prophylaxis of malaria, even in areas where *P. falciparum* is known to be resistant to all classical drugs (especially to chloroquine). Fansidar was marketed in 1970. Since then, research in the field of derivatives of the natural alkaloid quinine has led to a collaboration with Walter Reed Hospital. Walter Reed screens compounds from Roche, and Roche has done some new synthesis of Walter Reed compounds. This project has been considered by WHO and the responsible specialists of the Special Programme in Research for Tropical Diseases (TDR) as a first-priority project. Therefore, a collaboration between WHO, WRAIR, and Roche is progressing, and clinical trials are running in the three continents where malaria is a major health problem.

Research by Roche on schistosomiasis started twenty years ago. It reached the level of clinical trials in 1973, after thousands of compounds had been synthesized, and between twenty and thirty were found to have some desirable activity. The second screening was

14

carried out in Belo Horizonte (Brazil) and at the London School of Tropical Medicine for tests in monkey models and other animals. After these tests, the choice was narrowed to two compounds, with still more animal testing in several species. One of these was finally selected for clinical trials.

Roche is conducting major projects in filariasis and onchocerciasis in close cooperation with specialized research groups at universities. One of the basic problems is the absence of good laboratory models (substitutes for humans in testing) for these diseases. Still, the need for drugs in filariasis is so great that the company will continue its efforts. The company also has a small project in leishmaniasis, again cooperating with several universities, but it does not have a high priority, since the disease is not widespread. Work on leprosy has been limited to clinical research, involving sulfonamides and combinations of drugs.

Ciba-Geigy has had an effective drug (Ambilhar) in schistosomiasis since 1962, which is used in many countries of the Middle East, Africa, and Latin America (though in Brazil the drug is not effective against the *S. mansoni* strain). In malaria, the company had a program of testing compounds in monkeys for a number of years, but it achieved no success and was therefore dropped. The company has a useful drug against leprosy (Rimactan), and dosage tests are currently being made; it also developed Lamprene for leprosy, but it has a side effect of coloring the skin a reddish-brown tinge, which is slowly reversible; it is scarcely noticeable, however, in black skin.

The Wellcome Research Laboratories have worked in tropical medicine since 1913, concentrating on parasitic diseases. In 1940, they moved heavily into chemotherapy in tropical medicine, and have published over 1,000 professional articles in this field. Present interests include all but one of the six parasitic diseases—leprosy being excluded. A large amount of fundamental research underlies these tropical projects. Of the total Wellcome activities, 15 to 20 percent of the projects are in tropical diseases, or about $4 million of a $30 million total research budget.

The development of specific strains of the tropical diseases for laboratory testing is long and costly—the U.S. Army, for example, spent $11.5 million combating drug-resistant strains of malaria in Vietnam. At present, only two pharmaceutical companies in the world have malariologists, and Wellcome reported that both are now largely shifting out of malaria research. To conduct research in malaria requires maintaining six different animal species in the laboratory plus different disease strains for humans.

Wellcome has worked on schistosomiasis for thirty years and

found nothing, despite many promising starts. Research in leish-maniasis has also produced only little success; it remains costly to examine three animal species for three different disease forms. For trypanosomiasis, there is no good disease model, and there is no way to control the parasite carrier (vector), but the company is seek-ing to develop chemotherapy and immunology treatments for its control in both animals and humans. Filariasis is similarly a difficult research problem, which explains why there exist only two drugs for it. There is no adequate laboratory model of the disease.

Bayer has the longest tradition in tropical disease research among pharmaceutical companies. Suramin (Bayer 205) was discov-ered in 1916; it was the first effective drug against African trypa-nosomes and the only effective drug against macrofilariae, and it is still widely used. In the 1920s and 1930s malaria research was a very extensive part of Bayer's research program. These efforts led to the discovery of pamaquine (plasmochin), the first synthetic antimalaria drug, and to other very active compounds such as mepacrine (ate-brin) and resochin (chloroquine), which is still one of the most widely used antimalarials.

Against *Trypanosoma cruzi*, an intensive screening program was running from 1937 in which more than 24,000 compounds were included. Less than ten years ago chemotherapy of Chagas' disease was still an unsolved problem. Therefore, Bayer has intensified its activities in this field. Out of a very large series of compounds, especially synthetized for this indication, nifurtimox (Lampit) was found to be the most active. Through cooperation between South American and German scientists and clinicians, nifurtimox was tested experimentally and in clinical trials against a variety of *T. cruzi* strains infecting more than 1,600 patients. The clinical studies lasted from 1965 to 1973 in five countries; they were carried out under identical standardized conditions and controlled by an additional blind working reference laboratory. Basic knowledge on clinical fea-tures and serological and biological behavior of the parasites was obtained from those studies. In 1972 nifurtimox was introduced into the market as the first drug to treat the acute and the chronic phase of Chagas' disease. There are indications that nifurtimox is also suited for the treatment of the final stages of African sleeping sick-ness. The first findings in South America indicate that it is also effective against the mucocutaneous form of leishmaniasis.

After the successful work in Chagas' disease, the company shifted its resources to schistosomiasis, which has been given a top priority within tropical medicine. The aim was to develop a new antischistosomicidal drug effective against all strains of all schisto-

16

some species pathogenic to man after a single or a one-day treatment; at the same time it had to be well tolerated and thus suited for a population-based chemotherapy of schistosomiasis. Together with E.Merck/Darmstadt, Bayer started a very intensive research program about ten years ago.

These efforts led to the discovery of entirely new chemicals of the pyrazinoisoquinoline type. Praziquantel was found to be the most promising compound with respect to spectrum and intensity of activity, as well as tolerability. After finishing the evaluation of the efficacy of praziquantel against a variety of strains of all pathogenic schistosoma in various animal species, in cooperation with the London School of Tropical Medicine and Hygiene and the Schistosomiasis Research Unit in Belo Horizonte, clinical tests were started on a multinational basis. Intensive clinical trials in Zambia, Japan, and the Philippines, in a close cooperation with WHO in Brazil, confirmed the broad spectrum of activity and the excellent tolerability of praziquantel in human schistosomiasis. When praziquantel is made commercially available in the near future, it will fulfill most of the criteria of an ideal antischistosomicide and be well suited for a population-based program of chemotherapy. This success with praziquantel follows a long tradition in schistosomiasis, which also produced fuadin, lucathone, metrifonate, and bayluscid—a powerful molluscicide. (In addition, praziquantel is highly effective against other treatodes, such as Paragonimus and Clonorchis species, and against a variety of tapeworm species, as well as cystercosis.)

Bayer also has a project in filariasis and onchocerciasis. There is still a great need for an effective drug in these indications. After the new compounds have passed the first screening in two rodent-models, they will be tested in some of the WHO filariae centers in Germany, the United Kingdom, and Australia against various filarial species in different host animals. At present, there are some promising new experimental drugs under intensive investigations. One of them is amidantel, a new anthelminthic, which is also in clinical trials for use against hookworm and ascaris infections in humans.

Hoechst has been working on drug compounds for malaria and filariasis, though commercial opportunities are virtually nonexistent. To meet its costs it has applied for grants from the German Ministry of Research and Technology as well as WHO and has received small support funds. It has succeeded in developing a compound for malaria, which it is currently moving into the developmental phase, but the compound will not be fully tested for five or six years. Its program on filariasis is simply a screening project under the WHO grant.

Results for Six Diseases

Despite a long period of research in tropical diseases by a number of companies, there are still gaps in the protection against the six diseases selected for WHO's Special Program. The usefulness of each drug was assessed by different company researchers during the interviews as follows:

Schistosomiasis. Hycanthone (by Sterling-Winthrop) appeared to be promising because a single dose was active against both intestinal and urinary schistosomiasis. Unfortunately, it is costly and has been found to be mutagenic and possibly carcinogenic in some animal tests. Bilarcil (Bayer) is an organophosphate that has been widely used in Africa; doses must be taken two to four weeks apart, but it works on only one type of schistosomiasis (*S. haematobium*).

Ambilhar (Ciba-Geigy) requires daily doses for five to seven days. A psychotic reaction is sometimes a problem, and the drug appears to be probably carcinogenic in animals. There have been rare reports of liver damage. Oxamniquine (Pfizer) works only against the intestinal form (*S. masoni*) and appears to be safe and inexpensive for the single doses needed. The African species of *S. mansoni* appears to be less affected by the drug; therefore, repeated doses are required, which makes it too costly and difficult to administer. Praziquantel (Bayer and Merck/Darmstadt) seems to fulfill most of the criteria of an ideal schistosomicidal drug. In clinical trials, this new compound was shown to be effective in an oral, single or a one-day treatment against all schistosome species parasitic in man and was well tolerated. It is not yet marketed, however.

Filariasis. There are two drugs: Diethylcarbamazine (DEC), marketed in 1948, is the more useful, but it may cause complications such as shock when patients are heavily parasitized. Some $20 million has been spent by various groups in trying to improve its use in the field. The second drug, suramine, is considered to be toxic and requires seven weekly intravenous injections. Therefore, there is no satisfactory drug, as yet. It is difficult for researchers to close the gap, though work is still progressing. Ciba-Geigy is researching certain new compounds in an effort to meet the criteria of the WHO Special Program.

Malaria. Quinine at one time had been superseded by other drugs, but parasites eventually developed resistance to the new drugs, and quinine is back in favor, although it is relatively toxic. Chloroquine often cures disease or suppresses its development; it is inexpensive, but causes some minor side effects. Chloroquine-resistant strains have arisen in Vietnam, Thailand, Indonesia, and the Philippines, and recently in Burma, Bangladesh, Northeast India, and Nepal. In South America, *P. falciparum* did not respond to quinine or chloroquine.

It would appear that new chemical types are needed to avoid the crossover of resistant strains that are keeping the disease prevalent. Many companies all over the world have contributed to the research efforts of the U.S. WRAIR. Some analogs of new drugs tested by the U.S. Army were also treated by firms such as Wellcome. As noted above, Roche is contributing to the development of Fansidar and of quinine derivatives, especially mefloquine, in close collaboration with WHO and WRAIR.

African trypanosomiasis. There has been no breakthrough in chemotherapy in the last twenty years. Pentamidine isothionate is still used, though resistance may occur. Melarsoprol is active, but very toxic.

American trypanosomiasis (Chagas' disease). This form became a curable disease a few years ago, with the introduction of Lampit and Radanil.

Leishmaniasis. There are a limited number of drugs. For thirty years, Wellcome has had Pentostam, which is considered to be the drug of choice. The incidence of the disease is small, making the market small and providing no stimulus to company research for other drugs. After dropping research on this disease ten years ago, however, some companies have begun it again because WHO has included it in its Special Program. Consequently, R & D budget discussions in several companies have focused on "program gaps" to see if they are meeting future needs.

Leprosy. Besides the older sulfone derivatives and a series of long-acting sufonamides, new drugs are being studied: Rifampicin (called Rifampin in the United States) is available for treatment and marketed by Lepetit (Rifadin) and by Ciba-Geigy (Rimactan). Bacteriological and clinical research is going on to reduce the cost per patient by a less frequent application. Lepetit is working on a derivative of the drug. Further emphasis is hindered by the restricted market—

19

only 20 percent of some 20 million lepers get any treatment at all because of poor distribution systems in leprosy endemic areas and higher priorities to other infectious diseases.

Company R & D Criteria

Although the pharmaceutical industry, as a whole, covers all six diseases, more resources and effort are required to reach the goals of the Special Program in Tropical Disease Research, which include quick development of new means of treatment. Given resource constraints, this would require a *shift* in resource allocations and a change in the application of R & D decision criteria in some companies.

The criteria used by companies to determine whether or not to pursue research on a given disease are not identical. They generally involve the following: (1) medical need for a particular drug; (2) market opportunities for its sale; (3) present capacities and capabilities of the company's laboratory, including those which it might acquire easily from outsiders under contract; (4) probability of success of the project (that is, its experimental feasibility including the existence of disease models); (5) cost of the project in money and manpower, and in the opportunity cost of dropping or not undertaking other projects; (6) extent of competition in the field; and (7) expectations as to government provision and enforcement of patient protection.

On the basis of its assessment of these factors, one company interviewed had decided not to go into tropical disease medicines at all. It concluded that there was sufficient competition in the field, that the probability of success was low, and that market opportunities in some of the diseases were nonexistent. Another company dropped out of malaria when its compound failed in monkeys, but it has since been working on dosage designs and forms of other drugs for malaria. The few compounds Walter Reed Hospital has found for malaria have been followed up by only one company, which has a capacity to handle a complete range of drugs. (Only Roche, Ciba-Geigy, Rhône-Poulenc, and Bayer reportedly have such a capability, giving support to the assertion that only large companies have facilities in research and clinical testing to bring complex compounds through development into drug form.)

Another company has decided to stay out of malaria research because the chances of achieving any success in that field do not warrant substantial outlays of funds or manpower. Instead, out of a total of 4,000 compounds it develops, the company sends some

2,400 each year to Walter Reed Hospital. It is the view of this company each year that the small attention paid by pharmaceutical companies to leprosy reflects the disease's low social priority. Although leprosy is difficult to cure, it is not readily communicable and, therefore, not very dangerous to the community. One company decided not to do anything in leprosy because it could not grow the necessary bacteria (leprobacillus) readily in animals and because it was not engaged in TB research, which provides some potential synergy with leprosy research.

Another company ran into profitability problems during the early 1970s and cut back on its research, eliminating entire areas of activity—including chemotherapy and parasitology, veterinary medicine, and anti-inflammatory drugs. Concentration on what the company considered to be better market opportunities precluded continuation of its work in schistosomiasis, which had been both complex and frustrating. The company had tested a schistosomicide in Puerto Rico, with apparently positive results; then it found that the worms in humans produce eggs only periodically and that low egg production was being interpreted mistakenly as an indication that the drug was effective.

Another company doing virtually no work on the six diseases reported that it was unlikely to do so in the future simply because it cannot get an adequate return on sales to cover costs of development. A serious limitation to its interest in the developing countries is the necessity to establish clinical facilities, which were considered too difficult to set up and too expensive.

Among those companies doing research, most specialize among disease types or areas of fundamental research, thus precluding efforts in rather different areas of one or more of the tropical diseases. Several of the companies have decided that their research capabilities are already stretched beyond the optimum, which means that any new activities will have to be offset by dropping others. R & D requires not only professional personnel but also support personnel, physical equipment, and most importantly research management. Managers of R & D labs are generally selected from among the company's professional scientists, which means that some of the most successful researchers are pulled off of projects for administrative positions. Since their training is seldom in management tasks of budget allocations, personnel management, or committee communication with other functional areas of the company, personnel with the required capabilities are scarce. Management is made more difficult by the long lead-time in resource commitment prior to research results—as long as ten years for discovery of useful compounds. In addition, the time lag between initial drug discovery and marketing is between ten and twelve years: five years for drug development, another two to five for completion of preclinical and clinical trials, plus toxicity testing and one or two years for premarketing studies. A total period of around twenty years from initial concept to marketing is not unusual. This long gestation time makes for long turnaround times among R & D projects, unless failure is recognized at the early stages. It makes planning difficult and reduces the capacity to introduce new projects because resources are committed long-term.

Among the project decision-criteria, three related to markets are required before any company is likely to support work on a given disease: (1) the disease is significant in worldwide health needs and demands; (2) there are marketing possibilities in most areas where the company operates, not merely in limited markets of a few countries; (3) potential users of the drugs (for tropical diseases, this means mostly governments) are able and willing to buy. This point was stressed by an official of Wellcome at the 1974 WHO/industry conference in Paris:

> It is, perhaps, important to bring the situation into practical perspective. Basically, industry is not faced with a problem but rather with a dilemma over choice to invest in programs with hitherto poor financial return or to concentrate their resource allocation to more obvious sources of reasonable reward. This is a conflict between humanitarian outlook and the basis of economic viability. In contrast, the problem lies in the developing countries themselves and with those international or national institutions vested with the responsibility and the basis for incentive to promote the well being of the peoples of these countries. Solution to the difficulty is likely to arise only if the essential requirements of industry are recognized and means found to meet them satisfactorily. Indeed, it could be that the greatest incentive to industry for investment in this field would be evidence of obvious intent to utilize drugs already developed and at a level which would indicate the prospect of reasonable return on potential future development.[8]

If the three criteria are met, any company will try to develop the capacity to perform appropriate R & D even to the point of buying expertise from independent laboratories. Companies respond to market pulls, which are weak in tropical countries. Thus, additional

---

[8] O.S. Standen, "Preclinical Development of Drugs," in M. Marois, ed., *Chemotherapeutic Agents*, p. 216.

public programs are needed to fund the purchase and application of drugs in LDCs. Where companies see overriding sociopolitical or sociopsychological obstacles to government funding and mass distribution, they will not readily devote R & D projects to tropical diseases.

Still, pharmaceutical companies do conduct research in diseases or health problems where the market is not strong or extensive, if they consider the problem itself important in providing research synergy or future breakthroughs. This is the case for some of the six diseases and for many not among them. But the determination of which diseases are important enough depends on whether the company has the capability of conducting research on them. If so, and if there is a research "fit" with other projects, the company is likely to pursue the project, even when expected profits are small. When a company has a specific capability in a problem area, researchers will press use of their expertise to "see if something can be done." In addition, many companies feel a social responsibility to contribute where possible to meet health needs.

Activities like this are affordable only by a company working on a large number of projects that allow "losers" to be supported by "winners" or in which synergy arises so that a loser in one area leads to a winner in another. Even for larger firms, the long period required to determine whether a compound is a loser means that large resources are tied up, and proposed research in tropical diseases cannot be undertaken. A few companies stated they would maintain R & D in these diseases despite commercial pressures; but if still greater pressures on R & D allocations arise, cuts will have to be made in some existing programs. However, for reasons of morale, it is often difficult to pull researchers off a project—even though its continuance is commercially unjustified. Sometimes, too, diseases that were thought to be eradicated reappear or crop up in other areas, requiring *new* projects instead of the less expensive modification efforts on existing drugs. An offsetting pressure, encouraging work in tropical diseases, is that companies wish to gain support for sales of other drugs in LDCs, which buy one-fourth of the world's pharmaceuticals. The companies would like to meet total health needs in LDCs, thereby showing their contribution to raising labor productivity and to stimulating economic growth in the developing countries.

In seeking to meet the needs of LDCs, a conflict arises between company and government criteria. The company is looking for a drug which is patentable, and governments seek a generic drug. If the drug is easy to produce and not patentable, public health systems of LDCs will turn to suppliers who can sell it cheaper because they have not borne the R & D costs—as, for example, Poland. The pharmaceutical companies are frequently not interested in nonpatentable drugs, but host governments are very much interested in them, so as to reduce cost of mass treatment.

Despite these differences, one R & D manager's personal assessment of the likelihood of finding appropriate drugs for the six diseases was cautiously hopeful:

1. The successful pursuit of an ideal compound for malaria would be profitable for companies already in this area of activity; success is likely to require better vector control as well, though reduction in use of pesticides has increased the incidence of malaria recently.

2. Some forms of schistosomiasis are already being met by chemotherapy; others will require further drug development, and ideal agents may well be found. However, drug programs must be combined with adequate vector control, which is not yet feasible.

3. Pursuit of an ideal drug for trypanosomiasis is commercially sound if a drug successful in animals could also be used for human disease control.

4. Leishmaniasis is widely dispersed geographically so the costs of its cure need not be borne by a single government; if an ideal compound could be found, it would probably be profitable.

5. Filariasis is probably too difficult to control with one drug because of the six different insects and types involved in this disease; it would require several drugs and, therefore, large R & D efforts.

6. A new drug for leprosy is not commercially viable; too few people are infected, and even with a new drug it would be too difficult to treat them under present conditions.

To achieve agreed-upon goals in controlling these diseases, several companies stress the need for better methods of setting priorities, based on cost-benefit analysis of the impacts and treatments of the six diseases. This would require determination of the quantitative and qualitative impacts of not controlling the diseases versus the costs and benefits of control. Complete eradication would be the objective for some of the diseases—such as malaria, which raises absenteeism from jobs, causing loss of production (which can be quantified), and which destroys brain tissues, reduces physical capabilities, and causes eventual loss of life, which cannot be valued in money terms. But the costs of total eradication are enormous, and developing countries will probably not have sufficient funds for such a program.

Immunology Approaches

In the hope of reducing significantly the administrative and delivery problems in disease control, the WHO Special Program has emphasized the approach of immunology (the use of a vaccine which provides immunity to the attacks of the parasites) over chemotherapy. Obviously, a single-shot vaccine against any of the diseases would be highly desirable, but creating such a vaccine is one of the most complex tasks in drug development. None of the companies interviewed considered it likely to be accomplished in the near future—although a vaccine for malaria may be only five to ten years away. Many of the companies are involved in vaccines and immunology, but they have not been assigned a high priority, largely because of the high cost and uncertainty of this approach.

Janssen is seeking immunization methods against several parasitic diseases by stimulating the development of natural antigens in the host through controlled injection of the parasite. The development of natural antigens could then provide immunization. One problem in this approach is timing: the parasites must be killed by the antigen before they can harm the patient. Some officials believe that antigens may be successful against certain types of worms—blood flukes, for example—but they are not certain about others. The problem is to find a chemical that can paralyze the parasitic invader and keep it in one spot so that the body can then mount its counterattack.

There is some evidence that individuals may gain immunity to some of the tropical diseases; those with sickle cell anemia, for example, have some immunity to malaria. However, it is difficult to develop a vaccine against invaders such as worms, which are complex, multiple-cell attackers. New discoveries in fundamental biology and chemistry are needed to find out how the attackers work and how to prevent their destruction from destroying other cells in the host. For vaccines against worms, what is needed is fundamental biochemical research on the worms themselves, rather than trial and error testing through simple procedures. A complex and interrelated scientific process is required, which can only be broken up at great cost.

Even for malaria, several problems complicate the process of discovery: (a) test cultures must be grown, but many cultures are stable only for a few days; (b) there are multiple strains and species of the disease, requiring multiple cultures; (c) immunization is not necessarily long-lasting in parasitic diseases; and (d) it is not certain what cells of the parasite should be attacked by a vaccine—that is, what part of the parasite actually causes the infection. Without knowledge of the precise process of the disease, it is difficult to specify what is to be immunized against.

Immunology projects to obtain such knowledge are high-risk and long-term because companies have reached the limits of applicability of their knowledge. New scientific understanding must be achieved and basic techniques must be developed to achieve a breakthrough. (This should explain why statements that companies are doing less and less may reflect the tracing of observed facts to incorrect causes.)

Ciba-Geigy has begun a program in immunology that may lead to novel therapies for malaria and other parasitic diseases. The project is being conducted in cooperation with a university in England and an industrial laboratory in Germany that specializes in vaccines. Testing in humans is several years away.

Roche has an institute on immunology, encompassing sixty specialists, engaged in basic work on vaccines. It has also financed an institute on molecular biology in New Jersey, concentrating on basic research and antiviral medicine (yellow fever, smallpox). Such basic knowledge is also necessary for further progress in immunology.

The Wellcome Laboratories have worked in the area of vaccines for several years and have developed some which are effective, for varying time periods, against viral and bacterial infection. The company considers its work on immunology as an "act of faith," likely to lead to considerable financial losses even if a vaccine is found. Commercial losses will occur because the vaccines can be readily duplicated and are not easily patentable because they are biological rather than chemical entities. Tropical countries would try to force the prices down for mass use, making production too unprofitable to recover development costs.

According to Wellcome scientists, one of the main problems in developing vaccines is the inability to obtain antigens. Worms cannot be reproduced in a culture; they are available only from animals, which makes their development and acquisition costly compared with lab-cultures, and animal antigens cannot be used in the lab to attack the worms. Some protozoa (such as those in Chagas' disease) can be started in animals and then multiplied in cultures. But, in the main, useful parasitic antigens are found only in the blood cells of the human hosts; these must be gotten out, studied, and then duplicated for production.

Permanent immunology has been found for no parasitic disease in humans; immunity is lost when exposure stops, even for malaria.

In some diseases, the degree of immunity that may exist in the human host cannot be determined. Does the body reject the parasite, or reduce its growth or gestation, or merely counter the ill effects of the invasion? Although it is known that some immunity can be built up against schistosomiasis, it is not known how or how much. Two prospective vaccines have been developed from injection of larvae into cows and dogs, but keeping the larvae alive has proven difficult.

Major difficulties arise from the inability to see even the theoretical applicability of vaccines in general—let alone any specific vaccine—to some of the diseases. Some researchers consider that the six tropical diseases will not yield to vaccines because the antigens will cause the parasites to develop resistance while in the body and develop a new strain of the disease, as has happened with influenza. It appears that malaria and possibly Chagas' disease would respond to vaccines, but tests in animals show that the desired result must be stimulated by adjuvants, which may be irritants, and possibly carcinogenic. To reduce some of these effects will require vaccines from killed microorganisms rather than live ones, but "dead" vaccines are often not as effective as needed. Further problems arise in the attempt to use blood cultures from tropical countries, which must be tested for many other diseases before they can be used for the production of the culture of the disease under study.

Since malaria seems to be the most likely candidate for a vaccine, Wellcome has been working on it, as have Rochester University and Walter Reed Hospital. But Wellcome considers that the worst policy would be to rush into field trials before it conducts careful clinical trials, which will not occur before 1985. Field trials will take an indefinite period, and the difficult task of scaling up for production of the vaccine will also take time. In addition, Wellcome managers are not sure that acceptable adjuvants are available, nor are they sure that the vaccine will work when the patient is already infected, as in the case in parasitic diseases where repeated infection occurs. Nor do they know whether infants can be inoculated. Wellcome already has a scientist and technicians working on the malaria culture problems, plus other professionals working on the problems of batch culture processes and chemists on the adjuvants. The company's manpower commitment will increase in the next several years as it moves toward clinical trials.

One of the European countries noted that research in immunology in both Europe and the United States has been confined largely to public health-related institutes—for example, the Pasteur Institute in France and the U.S. National Institutes of Health—both producing their own vaccines. Private companies have been afraid of liability suits of the sort that arose in the case of the Swine Flu Program in 1975. In addition, when the federal government in tropical countries requires vaccinations, public health institutes are the units that implement the program, and the companies cannot be certain that appropriate procedures will be followed.

Other Resources on Diseases in Developing Countries

Pharmaceutical companies have made commitments to the needs of developing countries in areas other than the development of drugs for the six parasitic diseases. Many LDC diseases of significance earlier—for example, smallpox and yellow fever—have been successfully treated by vaccines and chemotherapy. The consequence has been to raise the six tropical diseases to a greater relative importance. The work of many companies on advanced-country problems has had beneficial results in developing countries. Among these health care problems, as seen by some R & D managers, the most important is that of fertility. In a second group fall respiratory problems (TB, in particular), along with tetanus and eye, ear, nose, and throat infections. At a third level fall intestinal diseases (parasitic or not), cholera, measles, epilepsy, diabetes, and skin and venereal diseases; and the least pressing is trauma from shock. WHO itself includes hypertension among its health priorities for LDCs—stemming from reactions to urbanization, industrialization, and the breakup of extended families.

All of these are subjects of research by the pharmaceutical industry. Indeed, LDC health problems are beginning to match patterns in advanced countries. But not all experience in one is directly transferrable to the other. For example, Ciba-Geigy has an anti-TB drug (Rimactane) which proved highly effective. It is easily affordable in the advanced countries, where dosages are sold for $1 per day for a year's treatment. After about a month in a sanitorium, treatment can be continued at home. Since sanitoriums are relatively expensive in developing countries, ambulatory (at home) treatment is highly desirable. The drug shows promise in LDCs.

The company selected Indonesia as an area for field trials of the drug, in response to requests by the Indonesian government and consultation with WHO officials. Some 4 million cases of TB exist in Indonesia, making the disease second only to malaria, and it is poorly controlled. In 1975, the government included an anti-TB program in its five-year plan; the Ministry of Health, Ciba-Geigy, and doctors in the field cooperated in this project. Its purpose was mainly to determine if the drug afforded more simple and practical treatment of TB than that using streptomycin, which had a long treatment period, high dropout rates, and a lack of patient interest and follow-up. The results on a six-month and a nine-month regimen combining Rimactane with other drugs were compared with prior treatments. Total coverage in the trials included 300 patients in government TB centers at Malang and Bali. Evaluation of results were closely monitored by modern methods, that is, by computerized programmers and sputum analysis locally and by an international laboratory in the United Kingdom. The results were very encouraging, and the Ministry of Health decided to use these regimens for larger projects to gain more experience and control under a suitable health care infrastructure. The results are again encouraging. The short course therapy with Rimactane has opened up practical new ways to eradicate this disease. However, large-scale eradication programs will eventually depend on support from the highest levels in the government, providing financial resources and health care organizations. WHO could extend assistance to these efforts based on its experience in other countries.

Roche also has developed several drugs to treat TB, but different dosage forms and delivery systems will be required for the third world. Some of the drugs are too expensive for mass distribution. Roche has also marketed drugs for intestinal parasites—tape worms and round worms—with which millions of people are infected. Over the past five years the company has developed drugs that remove 80 percent of these worms from a human host.

Roche is working in other areas of interest to LDCs also, for example, on amoebic dysentery and several bacterial diseases—cholera, bacterial dysentery, and typhoid. It has produced a drug (Valium) which has been useful in reducing tetanus in children, caused by the cutting of the umbilical cord, piercing of earlobes, circumcision, and accidents. Tetanus has been the largest killer of children in some African states. This drug works even after convulsions have set in and the disease is at an advanced state. The company has also developed a drug useful against epi-meningitis and cholera. The drug is stored by WHO in case of epidemics, but since it has a shelf life that is often less than the period between epidemics, the company buys back the stocks that have been stored too long, which makes the company's operations rather costly.

Another pharmaceutical company has been in controversy with WHO on development of a long-lasting injectable fertility drug. But WHO's safety standards are similar to those of the U.S. Food and Drug Administration (FDA), which will be difficult to meet with an injectable drug. However, WHO does not require the same standards of *efficacy* as the FDA, since it considers that even 50 percent effectiveness would be an improvement over present fertility rates. To protect against side effects and toxicity, WHO has promised to support toxicity trials in animals (rodents, dogs, and possibly primates) over a two-year period. These trials will probably take place in an independent lab, since the company would not want to commit programs of its own resources to a single activity of such magnitude, given competing claims on personnel and facilities.

A problem for oral preventives in many of the LDCs, is that the women will not take the antifertility pills regularly. This has made it difficult to obtain scientifically satisfactory results from clinical trials of oral drugs, which must be conducted locally to determine if there are differences among inhabitants of different regions or countries. These problems have caused WHO to emphasize an injectable drug. The company does not anticipate great differences in the pregnancy chemistry of women around the world and, therefore, in the efficacy of the drug, but the side effects could well be different. Extensive trials will be needed.

Parke-Davis is doing considerable research in areas of interest to the developing countries outside the six special diseases. It has marketed three drugs for intestinal helminthiasis; two for amoebiasis; one for herpes infections; fourteen for typhoid, typhus, cholera, tetanus, and other bacterial diseases. One vaccine for influenza and two each for measles and poliomyelitis have been developed. And, since the company had some overcapacity in its R & D lab, it has done $1.1 million of contract work for the Agency for International Development (AID) and other agencies on malaria, measles, and some vaccines for the period 1976–1977, to which it contributed $0.4 million as part of the overhead cost.

Pfizer's work in anthelminthics for veterinary medicine is also useful for human diseases. And its specialization in antibiotics will be useful in inflammatory diseases such as trachoma.

Janssen is working on broad-spectrum anthelminthics and hopes to market the drugs through affiliates of Johnson & Johnson in various tropical countries. The lab has given its first priority to anthelminthics largely because of the interest of a chief researcher, who is a professor of microbiology and parasitology as well as a veterinarian. After spending seventeen years in the tropical regions of Africa, he has concluded that it will be virtually impossible to change the personal hygiene customs of the people, meaning that they will be re-infected periodically so that removal of worms will require systematic treatment under the direction of health personnel. Janssen has developed a broad-spectrum drug which need be used only two or three times a year. The drug seems to be effective against many types of worms, expelling some 60 percent of the tapeworms. The drug is also effective against the guineaworm, and a higher dosage can control the Philippine worm. The company has been working with the U.S. Naval Research Unit in the Philippines for about a year on control of nematodes, flukes, and roundworms.[9] Janssen is also working on lamberia, using dogs to screen the drug. It has also conducted field trials of various drugs in developing countries; it tested for stomach cysts among nomads in Kenya, where some 25 percent of the deaths result from this disease.

Much of what Wellcome has done in tropical diseases has come through its efforts in diseases such as yellow fever, poliomyelitis, typhoid fever, and cholera. It is also working on anthelminthics, amoebiasis, and tropical veterinary medicine. Its veterinary research concentrates on cattle diseases, since the continued upgrading of cattle in LDCs will increase the animals' exposure to disease. The company is also studying diseases in sheep and means to control vectors such as ticks, flies, and mosquitoes; an experiment in the Middle East will focus on fly control.

Bayer is working on broad-spectrum anthelminthics and is developing a new drug against hookworm and ascaris (roundworm) infectious in man. Its work in veterinary medicines concentrates on ruminant helminthic diseases, including cysticercosis. Bayer has also a major program on fungal disease and is generating some quite useful results.

Hoechst has concentrated on anthelminthics and antibiotics. It is also working on single-cell proteins in order to improve nutrition.

The contributions of pharmaceutical companies thus include substantial R & D resources committed to meet priorities in LDC health problems other than the six diseases. WHO's own budget allocation reflects priorities similar to those set by the industry for its research: the six diseases are "special" only within these larger goals, and three of them are considered minor. Although the companies are involved in the Special Program because the six diseases may yield to chemotherapy, the six differ from some health problems in that much more than an effective drug is needed. This is shown in chapter 4, on the Brazilian experience with schistosomiasis.

---

[9] T. C. Banzon, C. N. Surgson, and J. H. Cross, "Mebendazole Treatment for Intestinal Nematodes in a Philippine Barrio," *Journal of the Philippine Medical Association*, 52, 7–8 (1976).

3

Cooperative Activities

Pharmaceutical companies have gone beyond the business of developing and providing drugs in cooperating with laboratories, clinics, and public health authorities in programs of disease control. For example, Hoechst has cooperated with the Egyptian government in a program against schistosomiasis; Bayer has worked with the Bolivian government on Chagas' disease; and Pfizer has assisted the Brazilian government in a campaign against schistosomiasis, as discussed in chapter 4. Cooperative efforts include activities in research and clinical trials, training professionals for laboratory research, and supporting public health campaigns of control or eradication. WHO has encouraged such cooperation.

Cooperative Research, Screening, and Clinical Trials

Research. Efforts at cooperative research in developing countries are hindered by the absence of laboratories at the foreign affiliates of the international companies and by the scarcity of local laboratories in developing countries. Some governmental or independent laboratories do exist, providing the opportunity for joint research and clinical tests, in the environment where the drugs are to be used.

Some of the companies have undertaken specific cooperative research programs, such as that on trypanosomiasis by Pfizer in the former East African Union (Tanzania, Uganda, and Kenya). This program existed for over six years, until the breakup of the Union. Pfizer provided two or three professional researchers each year to the laboratory in Tanzania, in addition to some personnel from the Food and Agricultural Organization (FAO). In other countries, the company has instituted shorter-term cooperative programs on the conduct of field trials and has organized educational symposia for local medical technicians on the development of health programs—for example, it sponsored a forum on parasitology in the Philippines in late 1977. In Latin America, Pfizer employed regional medical consultants to organize educational programs for local medical and paramedical personnel. In Bangladesh, the company's medical staff assisted in the training of paramedical personnel for public health services.

Roche has developed cooperative procedures with universities and independent laboratories in Brazil for the screening and clinical tests of vaccines, which cannot yet be duplicated in African laboratories. Its local affiliate in Africa could assist in cooperative work, but most of the company's scientific work is too sophisticated to be carried out (even cooperatively) with foreign laboratories.

Because of its experience in Mexico, another company concluded that it is too difficult to set up cooperative programs with local research centers in LDCs. It considered R & D personnel there lacking in the educational orientation necessary to stimulate scientific creativity, even though some had been sent to the best European centers for training.[10] Long-term developments would therefore be required to achieve an appropriate scientific infrastructure for R & D in pharmaceuticals in many LDCs. However, Ciba-Geigy has established a pharmaceutical research center in India on diseases of developing countries, especially hookworm, amoebiasis, and filariasis. There are over 200 staff in the Indian center, excluding maintenance personnel. It has been successful in using hamsters for screening compounds against hookworms infecting humans.

Ciba-Geigy has placed a high priority on cooperative efforts in LDC agriculture, especially in the production of seeds and crops. Losses in LDCs from rodents, monkeys, mildew, and other factors are large, and the company has developed pesticides, fungicides, and molluscicides to cut the annual loss of 40 percent of crops resulting from insects, fungus, and snails. It has assisted in the development of a research group on cotton in the Sudan; insect swarms are tracked by radar so that the crops can be sprayed at the most appropriate time, reducing the damage.

In Brazil, Ciba-Geigy has supported an agriculture extension project that trains teachers to help increase productivity, to develop

---

[10] The need to popularize science and technology and inculcate a sense of curiosity and invention is recognized by leaders in science in many LDCs. Without it, the necessary personnel cannot be developed to staff the required infrastructure and build the science community. (See J.N. Behrman, *Industry Ties with Science and Technology in Developing Countries* [Cambridge, Mass: Oelgeschlager, Gunn, and Hain, 1980].)

hygiene in difficult environments, to organize buying and marketing co-ops, and even to assist in some preventive medicine. The government of Brazil funds and sponsors the program while Ciba-Geigy donates some of the infrastructure, some materials, and expertise. The role of the company was to "seed" the project so that it would grow on its own and multiply in other locations.

Hoechst has a cooperative research program in Brazil with the Instituto Oswaldo Cruz in Rio, a government institute, specializing on Chagas' disease. The program succeeded in developing a vaccine for the disease. Field trials have begun, and if successful, the drug will be produced by a new joint venture between the Brazilian Instituto and a Hoechst affiliate in Germany. Hoechst also has a cooperative program in South Korea on chemotherapy against helminthics (worms) that exist in Korea, Taiwan, and a few other Southeast Asian countries. Infections are often lethal, and no drug is available. The compound being developed showed toxicity in producing gallbladder lesions after a few months. Therefore, Hoechst dropped the program and gave all the information to the Korean government, which has moved into clinical testing; if the side effects can be contained, some ill health would be preferable to death.

Screening. Pharmaceutical companies engage in screening—that is, testing chemical compounds against a virus, parasite, or disease condition in vitro (test tube in a lab) or in animals—in cooperation with each other only on a very select and bilateral basis. It is usually done by companies or laboratories (independent or university) that have long-standing ties. Cooperative screening is difficult partly because each originating laboratory tends to use up all of the compound it makes in the various processes of synthesis. The company would have to make more compound for tests by others, at a cost of from $5,000 to $25,000 for each additional gram of compound. It is estimated that a single professional scientist costs up to $100,000 per year for salary and equipment, and it takes a considerable portion of his time to make a new compound in sufficient quantity for screening by others.

A drug company is also wary of permitting competitors to screen a compound if it has an interest in producing the resulting drug. If the originating laboratory has no such interest, it would be willing to permit another company to screen, and if the compound was a success, it would license the production. This aspect of the problem raises questions about WHO sponsorship of compound screening. WHO contracts include a clause permitting it to manufacture the drugs, even when the originating company wishes to manufacture—

that is, WHO takes an automatic license. This reduces the interest of the originating company in developing the drug.

Some company officials indicated that the most important qualities to seek in cooperative efforts are a dedication on the part of researchers to scientific truth and to adequate procedures to discover it. These attributes are especially important at the stage of clinical testing, where the protocols must be appropriate and complete and must be followed precisely.

In addition, there is a problem of secrecy and shared proprietary rights. Will the structure of the compound be disclosed to third parties (inadvertently or willingly)? Are there adequate rewards for the additional costs of cooperative projects? Despite these questions, some effective bilateral cooperation has occurred among companies not only through cooperative screening but also through joint research extending to clinical testing and into commercialization. Such cooperation is usually achieved by dividing the research along specific lines, rather than having all of the professionals working closely as a team on a particular compound or agent. Such cooperative work cannot be separated from manufacturing facilities or from other laboratory activities. If such a physical separation of activities is attempted, the projects tend to become irrelevant to the commercialization programs of the company and thereby lose its support. Companies are seldom interested in mere contract work for WHO or others.

Few companies have engaged in multilateral cooperation, because it has led to confused responsibilities and complex lines of communication. However, many of the companies asserted that they probably would undertake some multilateral cooperative efforts; synergy is necessary in the process of discovery, and the pharmaceutical industry is under pressure to justify its role around the world. The companies recognize that fulfillment of their social responsibilities will require new organizational structures to involve LDCs directly in R & D and to keep production costs within reason.

However, WHO's request for more extensive licensing of drugs among competitors runs into two major problems—the profitability of a drug manufactured and supplied by several companies, and the royalty return from open licensing. WHO would limit the duration of patent protection to encourage prompt and open production locally in LDCs. Limiting the royalties to the originators, however, decreases the incentive to license at all. Some company officials argued that a guarantee of five years of purchases by WHO or by governments would be more important to them than twenty-year patent protection. Patents are not secure against a challenge, and they are shortened in duration because of long developmental time. Also patents do not guarantee sales. So far, WHO has not resolved the problems of patent protection, licensing, or guaranteed marketing.

Clinical Trials. Several of the companies indicated that they expect to cooperate with WHO in clinical trials in some fields, but that such trials are difficult to conduct effectively. They require clear protocols, including precise criteria and methods of assessment, precise specification of what is to be solved, clear definitions of the disease being studied, and examination of the health of the persons participating in the trial. Records must be carefully maintained, and procedures followed precisely and without any change. This means that the whole process must be completely and carefully supervised. Any deviation at all will invalidate the test; but it is difficult to prevent changes when two or more groups are responsible. In multicenter trials, if one researcher changes the protocol, the results of all may be invalidated. In order to minimize these problems, when test runs are conducted in several countries, they should be controlled from a single center. Other difficulties arise from cultural and language differences, making it difficult to communicate precisely the identification or staging of the diseases and the interpretation of results.

Clinical tests in developing countries are made more difficult by the fact that many patients suffer from multiple diseases. Clinical trials for a vaccine or a drug require homogeneity among the patients, or controls for differences in their conditions. When vaccines are tested, for example, results must be isolated from the effects on one of the other disease conditions in *each* patient. Tests for doing this are available, but they are not yet used in field trials because of their difficulty and the expense of multiple screening of the patients, which requires regrouping them according to each of the diseases.

Cooperative Training for Research

WHO has suggested that the pharmaceutical companies give extensive assistance to cooperative training of scientists and technicians in LDCs, especially to cooperative research projects with government or independent laboratories in Africa, and that they help to establish new, locally run laboratories where needed. Some of the companies are engaged in these activities already; others are not.

Training in Company Laboratories. Wellcome has at least one person each year from the developing countries being trained in a laboratory or using its facilities. Commenting on the WHO proposal, however, one representative of the company said that African research institutes were less sophisticated than those in some other LDCs and lacking in personnel able to benefit from such training. Wellcome has discussed with WHO traineeships in malaria, immunology, clinical pharmacology, and quality control. Training outsiders raises questions of confidentiality, which the laboratory is careful to protect, and WHO has not yet developed a policy to provide adequate protection of laboratory developments revealed to trainees.

Another pharmaceutical company (one not working on tropical diseases) has helped train researchers from developing countries for several years. The company is not eager to open all its doors to outsiders, but it has trained persons in limited specialties (such as toxicology) and would do so again. Still, it is not eager to expand this type of cooperation significantly. Ten years ago it had several scientists from Egyptian and Indian governmental agencies. Such programs have not always succeeded in generating scientists for the developing country; when the programs lasted for more than a year the foreign scientists generally wanted to stay in Europe.

The three pharmaceutical companies in Switzerland (Roche, Ciba-Geigy, and Sandoz) set up the Basel Foundation on Tropical Diseases, to train young researchers and public health officials from LDCs. It has trained Africans for three to four months in programs given out in the bush, with the result that sanitation of the area has radically improved. The companies do not provide research training in Switzerland so that the trainee will not regard a sophisticated environment, which his country could not soon provide, as being necessary for research. The foundation considers it better to take the trainers to the local environment in the LDCs. This was feasible because of an oversupply of European doctors, who would go on such missions.

Several other R & D managers agreed that LDC technicians should be trained in their local environment, for the reasons stated above. One company has trained personnel from LDC government institutes to conduct quality control analysis on imported drugs. For example, it staffed and equipped a school for quality-control technicians in Indonesia with the cooperation of that government. After two years, it turned the operation over to the government, which is still running it under the direction of one of the former students.

Several laboratory officials asserted that drug development efforts should be separate from efforts to help train scientists. Given the urgency of the WHO Special Program, they considered that drug development should come first, with training being incidental to that process. New technologies will be needed for breakthroughs in drugs useful and safe in mass application before local health officials are trained in delivery systems.

The major Swiss companies have formed an association, known as Interpharma, which among other duties administers visits from outsiders and requests for training of technical assistants from LDCs. Over a two-and-a-half-year period (1975 through mid-1977) fifteen company visits were made by six individuals from Indonesia, India, Vietnam, Egypt, and Ethiopia. The officials of Interpharma also offered some training possibilities in laboratories of overseas affiliates of the member companies. These opportunities were included in a formal offer the Pharma World Association (IFPMA) made to WHO on training programs that members would undertake in line with the WHO Special Program in 1979. However, experience with trainees has shown that they have little power in their own country to accomplish what could be done, simply because they do not rank sufficiently high in the hierarchy of their health ministries. Therefore, most assistance to these personnel is never infused into the decision-making priorities of the health authorities.

Interpharma concluded that the developing countries do not place sufficiently high priority on health and health education. Few of the LDCs have an adequate public health infrastructure, and its development is greatly delayed because government expenditures for health average only a small percentage of national budgets. Other state activities, such as the military, receive much greater allowances.

An example of training technicians in their own environment is the work of the Swiss Capuchin friars in Ifakara, Tanzania, begun over fifty years ago to replace a mission which German Capuchins had established before World War I. Tanzania, then Tanganyika, had been mandated to Britain by the League of Nations after World War I, and the Swiss took over the work that their German brothers had conducted when the region was a German territory. From the 1940s on, the Swiss Capuchins assigned to East Africa received instruction in tropical medicine at the Swiss Tropical Institute in Basel, under the direction of Professor Rudolph Geigy.[11]

Professor Geigy was invited to undertake field research at Ifakara and was later offered facilities to set up a laboratory there. Facilities were built and were later run by Professor T.A. Freyvogel. He and Professor Geigy discussed the problems of Ifakara with the managing director of Ciba Ltd., who visited East Africa in 1959. As a result of

---

[11] R. Geigy, "Training on the Spot: Swiss Development Aid in Tanzania, 1960–1976," *Acta Tropical*, vol. 34, no. 4 (1976), pp. 290–306.

this visit, the six major chemical companies of Basel established a Basel Foundation for Aid to Developing Countries. This foundation sponsored the construction of a center at Ifakara to train aides for dispensaries and hospitals and to offer courses for students from the national medical school.

In the early 1970s the center shifted its training emphasis, when it became apparent that there was a need for medical workers more highly qualified than aides but not as highly trained as doctors. Roche, Ciba-Geigy, and Sandoz agreed to equip the school for its new three-year program and to turn over the school to the Tanzanian government in 1978. Of the required investment of around 1.6 million Swiss francs, 1 million came from the Basel Foundation, the remainder came from the Swiss government, the Capuchin Province, the Baldegger Sisters (another Catholic order), and the government of Tanzania. About 120 students make up its full student body; only one in ten applicants are accepted for training. The students perform daily assignments as medical assistants at the Capuchin St. Francis Hospital, in an area where trypanosomiasis is common. Constant contact with diseased persons lends relevancy and urgency to the classroom and lab work.

The training program is two-pronged, emphasizing improved sanitation to reduce exposure to tropical diseases, and protection against and identification of disease. The work at Ifakara has shown the feasibility of changing hygienic conditions, even in mud and mud-wattle huts, with such simple measures as care of drinking and cooking water, installation and care of toilets, careful storage of food-stuffs, opening smoke outlets and improving ventilation, protection against rodents, control of sand fleas, and use of mosquito nets. The second part deals with the specific measures to prevent or protect against multiple diseases. The trainee must be familiar with sixty-four tropical diseases—including quick worm, snail fever, sleeping sickness, and the plague—forty-four serious diseases plus some twenty minor ones. The students learn how to discover sources of disease in a community and then to protect against them with limited means. For example, they may study household sewage and refuse disposal and help build latrines in the community. In one instance, several cases of sleeping sickness were reported in the Serengeti National Park among the park staff and tourists. Staff and students from the center working with the East African Trypanosomiasis Research Organization (Uganda) discovered that hartebeests, lions, and hyenas acted as reservoirs for the disease, permitting the tsetse fly to pass it on to humans. Preventive measures were taken by the park staff.

During their studies, the students are required to spend six weeks out of the year helping in a cooperating village. Through the rest of the year they must pass an examination every Saturday morning in the classical courses of medicine—anatomy and physiology, pathology, pharmacy, and so on. Failure terminates their enrollment. Either immediately after graduation or later, the medical worker can obtain a position as the chief of a health center in a rural community. These centers provide more services than a rural dispensary, operated by a single medical aide, but fewer than a district hospital. Each center provides clinical services for up to 50,000 people and is responsible for all services concerned with prevention of disease and the promotion of health in the surrounding community. The center comprises the chief officer, nurses and midwives, a health education officer, a pharmacist, and an ambulance crew. Some 300 such health centers were projected for 1980, up from the 100 in 1977.

The success of this training for what amounts to general practice is attested by the fact that these aides, acting as the chief officers, correctly diagnosed and treated 90 percent of the cases they dealt with, as against 93 percent success for medical doctors in the country. The cost of training the aide is less than 8 percent of the cost of training a medical doctor and is six to eight years shorter. In addition, few of the doctors are willing to practice in the bush, where over 90 percent of the Tanzanian population lives.

All Swiss support will soon end, leaving a project which the Tanzanian government can continue without expensive overhead for buildings and equipment and without foreign assistance or management.

Establishment of African Laboratories. WHO is interested in developing laboratories around the world but has given a priority to Africa in the tropical diseases, since it contains all six. It seeks help in the creation of laboratories for drug development and support of clinical tests. Most of the companies interviewed recognize that it would be desirable to have laboratories near the diseases, but a number of problems exist. The first is an urgent need for competent researchers; training them is a long-term effort that cannot be shortened for medium-term development of drugs for the tropical diseases. The pharmaceutical laboratory at Endola, Zambia, was begun in 1977 using disease strains from cooperating companies on which to begin its research. However, it will, of course, need foreign scientists on the spot to train local scientists and technicians—one visiting professional for each four or five Africans to be trained in a three-to-five-year program. Expansion of programs such as this requires scientists from European industry, and this assignment may not be seen as useful to their careers. Nor is it certain that companies would donate the time of these professionals.

Companies consider that any LDC laboratory will require continuous and indefinite support from advanced counties (unless the LDC laboratory is narrowly specialized and has qualified leadership). Some company officials argue that training should begin at the universities, eventually with M.S. and Ph.D. level preparation, followed by laboratory training and still later by the establishment of a laboratory tied to production facilities, so that its work has commercial results. In such a sequence, the African laboratory would work on chemical entities developed by the universities and independent institutes, until it had gained sufficient expertise to develop its own compounds. Animal screening could then be added, followed by toxicological and clinical tests.

These separate processes in drug development are not mechanical but require independent thought. Difficult problems facing the new lab would be compounded by the long communication-distance (both geographical and cultural) of the research unit from other scientific communities. Efforts in the past were made to set up such research units in Cairo, Nairobi, and other locations, but they have failed for a variety of reasons, including restrictions on travel, language differences, difficulties of communication, and cultural differences. Some company officials commented that African laboratories would be under state ownership and control and that no new drug of outstanding significance has come from any state-owned laboratory; even after thirty years of R & D effort, the Eastern European pharmaceutical industry relies on drug development in western countries.

Given these problems, one official suggested that any specialized laboratory set up to work on tropical diseases should concentrate on the development stages between basic research and eventual drug production. It should *not* be located in Africa, he argued, but rather in Europe, where it would be close to the major research units and could maintain close ties with them. The laboratory would need some financing from WHO or other sources, but should have an independent management. A new type of institution would have to be created—separate from industry but tied to industry objectives. Problems would remain regarding the precise means of cooperation between this unit and industry laboratories. Would personnel be transferred from industry laboratories? What guarantees of markets would be provided for the products, and would there be a sharing of production among several companies? And, if such a center were established, would many of the companies now doing research on tropical new diseases reduce their research effort? Or would the new center work on applications of existing drugs within the African countries, helping to remove the obstacles to mass treatment?

Discussions with pharmaceutical companies about establishing laboratories in Africa on the six special diseases suggests that a substantial effort for at least ten years will be required before such laboratories could develop a drug to the state of application. The process itself summarizes the total R & D process in advanced countries, encompassing the same stages:

- Scientists and administrators must be trained—probably five years for scientists.

- There must be at least five professionals and five technicians for the examination of each of the six diseases in any country. Each disease has two or more forms, making fifteen to twenty specialized laboratories with ten persons each, or a total of up to 200. With the addition of an immunological approach, the number of personnel required could rise above 300. Adding the personnel required in animal screening (about 100) and toxicology (fifteen) brings the total to over 400 personnel.

- Clinical test capability would be required, involving numerous professionals and technicians over several years.

- Field trials would be required at several locations testing the drug against a specific type of disease and in various environments.

The time frame for accomplishment with little resource constraint is on the order of ten years if the entire program were planned in advance and the stages meshed—so that training and laboratory construction were done simultaneously, for example. Otherwise, disease priorities would have to be set.

One of the pharmaceutical companies has seriously considered offering to set up an indigenous laboratory and a production unit in Bangladesh. The company would obtain a return from exports of bulk items (compounding materials) to the foreign producer. Only if there is a satisfactory return, however, would the company be interested in such an endeavor. Further, the lab would not be useful without a tie to manufacturing. This particular proposal had not gone outside the company at the time of the interview, and was seen by top management as "idealistic" but "possible," reflecting an effort on the part of some officials in the company to see what might be done in a situation in which governmental interference and instability prevented normal business relations of investment or trade.

In sum, the views of the companies are that the establishment of African pharmaceutical labs would be difficult. Scientists oriented to industrial research cannot easily be developed outside of an industrial environment. And even though the existence of tropical diseases in the African countries makes research in certain diseases applicable and useful, a research environment is lacking. Nor is there an adequate delivery system for medicines and health care, which would stimulate local manufacturing and, in turn, require lab support at least in quality control.

Assistance in Delivery Systems

Only about 5 percent of the population in the developing countries is reached through doctors and pharmacists, who are the normal channels of drug delivery in the advanced countries. As is recognized in the WHO program and emphasized even more strongly by the pharmaceutical companies, a necessary component of the treatment of tropical disease is an adequate delivery system—especially in rural areas. The delivery system for drugs is based on two channels—through physicians in private practice and through various public health services sponsored by state, local, or federal governments. In the first, the use of the drug depends on the individual doctor's decision, and the distribution of the drugs depends on a network of warehousing and wholesaling activities under the control of the companies or the doctors. The development of this network would itself be a contribution of substantial value to LDCs which have not previously had such a network. But, in most developing countries, there is a lack of physicians, and those that exist are spread unevenly throughout the population. In addition, many of them are ignorant of the incidence of particular diseases in their localities since they see only patients who come for treatment.

Few developing countries have public health services as extensive as needed, and the progress of public health still relies significantly on individual physicians. Within public health programs that have been instituted, there is significant specialization on a few diseases, or even a single disease, leaving others unattended.

These limits seriously hamper the ability to deliver drugs to the areas affected by various diseases. In some cases, governments have refused to be the distributor (for example, contraceptives in Indonesia); in other countries, the same drugs are distributed through government-supported public health centers. In Africa, the government is the only purchaser. For most of the drugs for tropical diseases, the pharmaceutical companies are not involved in distribution through programs of disease control. This delivery gap is a serious problem in control of tropical diseases.

Pharmaceutical companies have assisted in campaigns against specific diseases or health problems, including assistance on food production and preparation, nutrition, sanitation, and education. A few have helped develop audiovisual materials designed to increase public awareness of worm diseases, through control by sanitation and other measures. Companies have also assisted government agencies by supplying personnel for the planning of a campaign against a disease and the training of technicians in the field. Some company personnel have been hired away by health ministries to help conduct such campaigns.

Techniques of education and promotion are useful in the developing country in other programs, such as pediatrics and prenatal counseling. They also contribute to promotion of self-medication by patients. But success in such promotional activities is much more easily attained when the disease is acute and the symptoms immediate; the concentrated attention of the patient is obtained causing him to "pull-through" the information provided. Unfortunately, the six tropical diseases develop so slowly that those infected are not induced to treat themselves prior to the appearance of acute symptoms. Motivation is weak because the direct tie between the drug and the disease is not evident.

One company is planning a program with Nigeria in the treatment of malaria, beginning with children up to five years old. Those between five and ten years with malaria will be treated in school, and those from eleven to sixteen will be treated only if there is a diagnosed infection. Pregnant women will be treated through clinics; other adults will not be treated at all in this particular exercise. Each province in Nigeria is to carry out its own part of the program, but technical development and administrative organization in each province varies greatly so that considerable company and federal assistance will be required.

Many of the companies considered that by far the largest portion of the responsibility for delivery of health care rested with the host countries themselves, who could turn to WHO and the companies for some direct and specific assistance. But, until the governments of developing countries altered their own priorities on health, little could be done by either the companies or WHO. To make this shift, LDC governments will need a better appreciation of what is required in developing an effective delivery system—and this recognition must exist at the ministerial level. Otherwise, the program will not get the funding it needs. The development of an effective delivery system requires training technical personnel, persuading these personnel to adopt a high level of dedication to the task (so as to carry it out precisely), educating the patients, and generating a "total program" orientation covering sanitation, vector control, education, and treatment, and creating the necessary administrative services. Few LDC governments have shown either the interest or the ability to adopt such an orientation. Without it, R & D efforts of pharmaceutical companies are less than fruitful, and their interest in continuing them will be dampened.

Two illustrations of how companies have cooperated in delivery systems are provided in the published literature related to schistosomiasis and leprosy. These are summarized below.

Schistosomiasis in Madagascar. In the area of the lower Mangoky in Madagascar, in 1966, the Samangoky Mixed Management Company was developing a vast irrigation system for the cultivation of cotton. The development of new water systems and the movement of new laborers into the region signaled the possibility that schistosomiasis would spread. At the initiative of Dr. Lambert, of the Ciba Laboratories, who had developed a new chemotherapeutic agent against schistosomiasis (Ambilhar), it was decided to conduct field trials in newly irrigated areas. Several groups combined to support and conduct the program: the government of the Malagasy Republic, its Ministry of Public Health and Population, the Technical Cooperation Service of the Swiss Confederation, the Swiss Tropical Institute, Ciba, and Shell International Chemical Company. Shell provided the molluscicide (Frescon) while the Malagasy government supplied buildings and some personnel and operating costs. Additional funding was provided by the Swiss Technical Cooperation Service, Ciba, and Shell. The project was conducted under an agreement with the Malagasy government covering a five-year period from 1966 to late 1971, when the project was turned over to the Malagasy government for its continuation.

The objective was to prevent introduction of the disease to the area through the new irrigation works, breaking the disease chain in two places: cleaning out the snails before the workers arrived, and eliminating infections in those moving into the region. Rigorously controlling the irrigation system and applying the molluscicide as necessary would eliminate the snails (intermediate hosts to the parasites) and reduce the chances that a transmission cycle would start.

However, two of the six subzones of the region, which were being treated, suddenly showed the existence of a transmission cycle, forcing both control and prevention activities to be undertaken simultaneously. The project was conducted under extremely difficult circumstances—poor supply channels, bad communications, major and uncontrolled migrations of workers, the flooding of the area three times by the Mangoky River, which increased the problems of snail control—along with administrative difficulties and cultural biases which impeded the effective administration of the program.

Despite the difficulties, the overall level of infection was reduced to around 4 percent of the population—a level of infection roughly corresponding to areas outside of the target region. This success was achieved at a cost of 23 Swiss francs ($7 equivalent) per person protected per year, including the costs of all equipment, vehicles, and buildings. The yearly costs declined over the program and were expected to decrease further in the consolidation period.

These results would not necessarily be duplicated in other countries because the disease treated was predominantly *S. haematobium*, one out of the three schistosomes causing the disease.[12]

Many of the problems in the project had less to do with drugs than with social and cultural conditions. The previous inhabitants of the area disliked the cotton company and the irrigation of the land, and they identified the medical technicians with this new enterprise, seeing them as "missionaries" sent to bother the inhabitants about sanitary problems, which they regarded as having little importance. It was necessary for the health technicians to show their independence from the company on several occasions in order to be able to gain acceptance and introduce education programs. The different ethnic groups in the area and the mixed population of tenant farmers and traditional farmers made the administrative structure difficult to set up, since many of the new inhabitants did not have an established community authority structure which could be used to get the message across. The administrative problems are made more difficult by inadequate public health service and the lack of coordination between the public and private health facilities.

The technical team estimated that the prevalence of schistosomiasis in the Samangoky area ranged from 10 to 15 percent at the beginning of the project in 1966. With the movement of workers and

---

[12] The description of activities and results of the project are given fully by A.A. Degremont, *Mangoky Project—Campaign against Schistosomiasis in the Lower-Mangoky* (Basel: Swiss Tropical Institute, 1973). See also "The Mangoky Project," *Journal of the World Medical Association*, vol. 5 (September/October 1975), pp. 65–69.

transients in and out of the area, conditions were ripe for an explosive increase in the disease, which, it was hoped, would be prevented by the following steps:

- systematic examination of the entire population and all immigrants to detect infections
- systematic treatment of all cases of schistosomiasis with niridazole (Ambilhar)
- inspection of all water in the area to locate snail habitats
- destruction of all snail habitats by chemical treatment (Frescon)
- establishment of sanitation facilities and health education programs, and inspection of new irrigation works
- definition of the scale of a subsequent, follow-on campaign and assessment of future costs of eradication.

Each technical team had to take a census of the inhabitants of its area because none was available and the populace moved so freely in and out of the area. The census procedure involved, first, a meeting with the leading citizens and inhabitants to explain that the census was solely for health purposes, since many were concerned about tax-gathering; then, painting of numbers on all houses; and finally, registering all inhabitants in each house. The census was updated every three to six months—consisting of a listing of new houses, registration of changes in the distribution of the population, identification of inhabitants not examined or treated, and preparation of a schedule showing the location and treatment of individuals. Even so, despite repeated efforts, it was difficult to track down all inhabitants.

Infection was determined by a urine analysis. Health cards were given to individuals if there was no evidence of the disease, or after treatment. Post-treatment checks were made one and two years after the mass treatment was started, so that patients treated in 1968 were checked every three months for the first year and then every year until 1971. Any treatment failures or reinfected patients were systematically retreated until the tests were negative.

Through health education, attempts were made to inform the people of the existence of the campaign and the necessity of treatment; dangerous areas of water were marked for the people to avoid. No effort was made to reduce contamination of the water with excreta, since a complete rural development plan would be required to alter habits and to provide better water supplies. Rather, the effort was directed at breaking the chain permanently by the removal of the snails and the considerable reduction of egg production in the human hosts. Efforts to obtain cooperation were supplemented by withholding monthly pay from those people not having up-to-date health cards and withholding cinema entertainment in villages where there were large numbers of latecomers or recalcitrants. The people then took communal coercive measures where necessary.

Extensive surveys of the snail population were made—including types of water and snails therein. Different techniques for eradicating the snails were required, depending on the terrain and whether the water was running or stagnant. Vegetation in the area of stagnant water made spraying of molluscicides both more difficult and more tedious than anticipated, since the spray failed to fall fully in the water. In some cases, in order to achieve desired results, water areas had to be cleared of vegetation, and recleared of recurring growth. Treating the waters required large numbers of workers and considerable amounts of chemicals and effort—not all of which would have been needed, the team concluded, if the irrigation project had been more carefully designed.

The malacological (snail) studies were made more difficult by exceptional flooding from the river. They were made still more difficult by the fact that the nature of the schistosomiasis in Madagascar appeared to be different from that on the African continent (though of the same type), making it impossible to draw on research or data from the latter. Numerous types of snails were found, and nearly 100 percent of some types were infested with *S. haematobium*. Different snail types were located in different bodies of water and required different methods of eradication.

Experiments were made in applying Frescon, at various concentrations, to determine the effect on the fish population in the various waters. The concentration necessary to kill snails destroyed all the fish, but fish returned through the flow of irrigation water after about fifteen days. During the time of treatment, fish floated to the surface dead or were stranded dying on the banks. The workers in the area gathered these fish for their tables despite warnings, but they showed no ill effects from eating the poisoned fish.

Over the five years, the project covered 23,228 people; 19,193 were examined and medical files were prepared; 4,035 people were left unchecked (17.4 percent). Of those unchecked, many were visitors staying in the area for less than fifteen days, some were new immigrants not yet contacted by the teams, and some were deliberately excluded from examination—infants under six months and the aged, blind, and crippled. Those excluded made up about 10 percent of the population, leaving only 7 percent which should have been included. Thus, something over 90 percent of those that should have been examined were treated. Given the increasing mistrust of the teams by the inhabitants, who saw them as representing the company, and given the large influx of temporary workers during the last year of the program, it would have been exceedingly costly to have reduced the number not treated.

The medication provided was distributed for seven days in a daily dosage of 25 milligrams per kilogram of body weight by a traveling team going through the villages. Team members watched to make sure that the medication was in fact taken. More than 9 percent of the cases of *S. haematobium* (the predominant type in the area) and nearly 29 percent of the much smaller number of *S. mansoni* cases developed relatively high intolerance to the drugs, shown in headaches and vomiting, with less frequent abdominal pain, dizziness, and muscular cramps. The ethnic groups in the region displayed notable differences in tolerance for the drug.

In assessing the project, the teams determined that one of the most important phases would be a follow-up with continuing health education for the people, including an improvement of sanitation conditions in the area. This would require both improved sanitation and a team of specialized, traveling teachers to explain health problems and their treatment. However, two years after the government took over, company officials reported after a visit that reinfestation of the area had occurred and that sanitation and health services were inadequate to continue with the necessary treatments.

Leprosy in New Guinea and Micronesia. In a series of trials in Karimui, New Guinea, and Micronesia, a sulfone drug developed by Parke-Davis was used against leprosy. Several articles have reported on the six-year experiments.[13] With the cooperation of a num-

---

[13] D. A. Russell, C. C. Shepard, D. H. McRae, G. C. Scott, and D. R. Vincin, "Treatment With 4, 4-Diacetyldiaminodiphebyl-sulfone (DADDS) of Leprosy Patients in Karimui, New Guinea," *The American Journal of Tropical Medicine and Hygiene,* vol. 20, no. 3 (1971), pp. 495–501. N. R. Sloan, B. Jano, R. M. Worth, R. Fasal, C. C. Shepard, "Repository Acedapsone in Leprosy Chemoprophylaxis and Treatment," *Lancet* (September 4, 1971), pp. 525–26. C. R. Broughton, G. C. Scott, D. A. Russell, and D. R. Vincin, "A Preliminary Report on the Use of the Depot Sulphone Preparation Acedapsone (Hansolar) in the Control of Leprosy," *The Medical Journal of Australia* (June 12, 1971), pp. 1258–63. D. A. Russell, R. M. Worth, D. Jano, P. Fasal, and C. C. Shepard, "Acedapsone in the Preventive Treatment of Leprosy," *Leprosy Review,* vol. 44 (1973), pp. 192–95. N. R. Sloan, R. M. Worth, B. Jano, P. Fasal, and C. C. Shepard, "Acedapsone in Leprosy Chemoprophylaxis: Field Trials in Three High-Prevalence Villages in Micronesia," *International Journal of Leprosy,* vol. 40, no. 1 (Jan.-March 1972), pp. 40–47. "Acedapsone in Leprosy Treatment: Trial in 68 Active Cases in Micronesia," Ibid., pp. 48–52. D. A. Russell, C. C. Shepard, D. H. McRae, G. C. Scott, and D. R. Vincin, "Acedapsone (DADDS) Treatment of Leprosy Patients in Karimui, Papua,

ber of schools and departments of public health, medical institutes, and hospitals, trials were quite successful. In one trial, the use of repository acedapsone once every seventy-five days for three years in some 1,400 individuals, who were both exposed to and susceptible to leprosy, led to a reduction of the number of new cases in the first year and to no new cases in the following year. In addition, sixty-six of the sixty-eight active cases treated improved satisfactorily during the three-year period.

The Ponape District of Micronesia was chosen for other field trials because leprosy had been prevalent there for nearly twenty years. Acedapsone (Hansolar, of Parke-Davis) requires no refrigeration and is therefore economical to administer in hot climates. It was given in regular injections to the entire population of three villages. Eleven new cases of leprosy were expected each year, but there were only six new cases the first year, and repeated examinations of the entire population in the subsequent two years showed no more new cases—thus only six cases arose, against an expected thirty-three, over the three-year period. No toxic effects were noted, nor any changes in the patterns of mortality or stillbirths.

The results of these trials indicated the possibility of mass treatment and eradication of leprosy; however, the effectiveness of the drug was tied to the prevalence of the disease in small villages with highly cooperative people. The experience does not indicate that the drug would be appropriate in large villages with low-prevalence of the disease.

The drug is injected only every seventy-five days, so it is preferred by patients and administrators to drugs that have to be taken orally twice a week. The absence of constant supervision made it impossible to know whether, in fact, the oral doses were taken. In the trial in Ponape, the infrequency of the injections kept down the costs of administering the drug. Only five professionals were needed on an intermittent basis to give the injection to nearly 1,500 people.

Another field trial in the Karimui area of New Guinea was set up in fourteen villages where the prevalence rate for leprosy ranged from 10 to 19 percent. Again, the results were highly favorable. The disappearance of skin lesions accelerated as treatment proceeded, and the highest cure rates were obtained in cases where treatment began immediately after an early diagnosis of the disease. This trial

New Guinea: Status at Six Years," *The American Journal of Tropical Medicine and Hygiene,* vol. 24, no. 3 (1975), pp. 485–95. D. A. Russell, R. M. Worth, B. Jano, P. Fasal, and C. C. Shepard, "Prevention of Leprosy by Acedapsone," *Lancet* (October 18, 1975), p. 771.

was begun in late 1967 and continued through December 1972. More than 460 patients were treated with acedapsone, with more than 95 percent receiving the injection at the prescribed intervals.

Leprosy had been diagnosed in most of the patients before mass treatment started, but a number of them had an inactive form and their condition did not change with treatment. This latter group was subsequently excluded from further analysis, leaving 269 patients with other forms of leprosy. And after five years of therapy, the disease was progressing or stationary in only 7 percent, and 93 percent were "healed" or "healing and improving."

The success of this project was significantly related to the fact that an injection was used and treatment was infrequent; the doctors concluded that "no other treatment could have been feasible in Karimui."[14] Frequent oral treatments would simply not have been accepted. Eradication of leprosy for a large population through the use of acedapsone as preventive treatment of all exposed people would require, however, a simultaneous and continuing control of all types of leprosy in that population in order to prevent reinfection and the need for continued treatment of individual cases.

---

[14] Russell et al., "Status at Six Years," p. 492.

4

Case Study: Schistosomiasis in Brazil

Schistosomiasis arrived in Brazil with infected slaves from West Africa, who were located in the Northeast, in humid areas where snails also live. The cycle of infection has more recently spread south and west through Brazil, as migration accelerated, to Brasília, the national capital in 1973 (see figure), and as far south as the State of Paraná.[15]

This chapter examines the Brazilian effort to control schistosomiasis which began over fifty years ago.[16] The recent program emerged out of an intense interest on the part of the government in the control of tropical diseases and a long-standing effort to establish adequate public health facilities throughout the country. Schistosomiasis had been given a high priority in these disease control programs for some years prior to the present program, but the drugs available were inadequate for mass control. New techniques and methods of control have been actively discussed for the past thirty or forty years. To control the snails, only calcium carbonate and a similar chemical were available, but they destroyed other life and damaged the ecological balance of the area. Even now, a sufficiently narrow chemical to control or eradicate the snails is not

---

[15] To determine the incidence of the disease, examinations of feces were conducted in 1975 along the trans-Amazon highway in the cities of Maraba and Altamira. Some 1,200 specimens were examined, with eighty-four (less than 7 percent) registering positive. All these positive findings were in the feces of persons from outside the region.

[16] This account is based on interviews at the Brazilian Ministry of Health, clinical laboratories in Belo Horizonte, the Pfizer laboratory in São Paulo, and visits to field operations in Natal in August 1977. In addition, three volumes of documentation provided by the ministry were analyzed (Ministerio da Saude, VI Conferencia Nacional da Saude, *Painel Programa Especial de Controle de Esquistossomose*, Brasília, vols. 1–3, August 1–5, 1977). Also examined was a series of articles on clinical testing of drugs for schistosomiasis and documentation for the program: "Symposium de Oxamniquine," *Revista do Instituto de Medicina Tropical de São Paulo*, 15, 6 (1973), pp. 1–176.

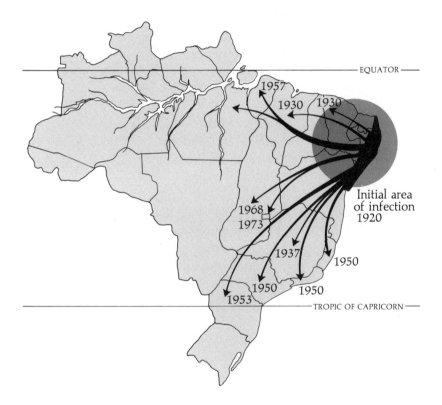

1957
1930
1930
Initial area
of infection
1920
1968
1973
1937
1950
1950
1950
1950
1953

EQUATOR

TROPIC OF CAPRICORN

SOURCE: Ministerio da Saude, VI Conferencia Nacional da Saude, *Painel Programa Especial de Controle de Esquistossomose,* vol. 1 (Brasília, August 1–5, 1977), p. 3.

available, since anything that will kill snails is dangerous to fish and shrimp.

The only drug available for treatment, beginning in 1918, was emetic tartar; for thirty years, from 1920 to 1950, two other antimonial drugs (faudine and astiban) could be used in humans but required at least a month of dosages and had bad side effects. In 1946, a new drug (lucanthone) arrived, but it also left much to be desired. By 1964–1965, two new drugs had been developed (niridazole and hycanthone), but were not fully launched until 1970. Both had undesired side effects, and hycathone faced problems in application because of the dosage form and the cost of follow-up.

In short, a mass program awaited availability of drugs that could be effectually applied on a large scale, and the planning process was tenuous and lengthy. Pfizer's oxamniquine was shown in trials to be successful but it would not have been adopted without prior screening and clinical tests by Brazilian labs.

Planning the Program

When oxamniquine was developed in 1970, the government was eager for a new and more useful drug, but another six years of planning and preparation were required before the program could be launched.

The Brazilian Minister of Health placed a higher priority on schistosomiasis because of his direct experience with the disease as a doctor in the Northeast area of Brazil. As workers moved into areas with large water bodies near the Amazon, the Ministry's Superintendency of Campaigns (SUCAM), which for years had been fighting a series of widespread diseases, particularly schistosomiasis and malaria, was catalyzed to mount a new, massive campaign on schistosomiasis. As a result, the health budget was raised progressively from 0.9 percent of the total federal budget in 1974 to 3.6 percent in 1977.

To plan the campaign, officials of the Ministry of Health went to conferences which Pfizer gave on the development and use of oxamniquine. The drug had been developed at the Pfizer laboratory in England and had undergone preclinical testing. It was later tested in Brazilian laboratories, which had been working on the disease. The officials remained quite skeptical, especially as to the dosage form, since they saw difficulties in using the original intramuscular (IM) dose in field application. They were also interested in the clinical tests undertaken in Brazil, but remained skeptical of what they termed "academic" results, having had difficulty using existing drugs in mass programs despite favorable clinical results.

Therefore, even though the clinical trials demonstrated the efficacy of the drug, the Ministry of Health conducted its own field trials to determine the effectiveness in field application. These field trials were the basis for the presentations to top government officials in justifying the mass program of control.

The overall program involves not just treating individuals with the drugs but also determining the locations for treatment, examining the populace, eliminating the snails, improving sanitation, and providing health education. The cost of the Brazilian program was greatly reduced by the fact that a public health system reaching into many rural areas already existed. This network not only made it much easier to determine how to go about the program but also meant that only marginal additions to personnel and resources in the field would be required, and that budgets could be kept lower and therefore would be more readily approved by the legislature.

The several parts of the program were projected to be synchronized so that snails would be eliminated at the same time drug treatment was given; the environmental sanitation and health education was projected to begin much earlier, so that people would be trained to act appropriately at the time of drug treatment. But it is not always possible to achieve such synchronization when there is a need to treat the populace and the movement of water continually floods new areas for snail breeding. The Ministry of Health, therefore, had to act against the disease without having previously eliminated the snails.

Animal Screening

Prior to this planning stage, Pfizer had engaged in screening oxamniquine in animals in Brazil, a significant factor in satisfying the Brazilian government. Several laboratories in Brazil had been testing alternative drugs for schistosomiasis in animals before 1970. A Schistosomiasis Research Unit (SRU) was officially established as part of the Institute of Biological Sciences at the Federal University of Minas Gerais in 1969. In addition, individual researchers at the university, attached to departments of medicine, parasitology, biology, and biochemistry, were working on various aspects of schistosomiasis. SRU tested the drug oxamniquine along with others that it had been studying. Pfizer provided the necessary supplies; tests were made by a forty-man group of professionals guided by a six-man supervisory committee.

The SRU laboratory is dedicated wholly to animal screening. At one time, it was doing nearly 10 percent of all screening of schistosomiasis drugs throughout the world—for companies such as Bayer, Beecham, Ciba-Geigy, Hoechst, Pfizer, Roche, Rhône-Poulenc, Wellcome, and Winthrop. The head of the laboratory, Dr. J. Pelligrino, had worked with each of these companies on an ad hoc basis, using compounds sent by them for screening in animals. The results of the laboratory's screening are returned to each company on a confidential basis, but in all cases the data have been published later.

Without these local research facilities, the schistosomiasis program would not have been accepted by the Brazilian government, for it wanted assessments of oxamniquine by its own scientists. The government also asked the opinions of many clinicians throughout the country on the work done at SRU. These doctors advised the government about the clinical tests and what they should seek in terms of field trials.

Clinical Tests

Clinical tests had also been conducted on oxamniquine by Dr. N. Katz, the head of a schistosomiasis institute, in Belo Horizonte. He developed an interest in schistosomiasis as a graduate student in 1963, at the Federal University, working with Dr. Pelligrino. Later, in 1965, in his own institute, Dr. Katz began clinical trials with niridazole and some other drugs. They produced side effects on the hospital patients and soldiers which would make them unacceptable for mass usage. (The results of these trials were not readily accepted by European and U.S. scientists, who could not believe that precise results could be obtained by work in Brazilian clinics. This attitude has now changed—according to Dr. Katz—and there is considerable beneficial cooperation.) The funds for these clinical trials of various drugs came from several international companies.

The research on oxamniquine was stimulated by a visit in 1968 of Drs. Pelligrino and Katz to the Pfizer lab at Sandwich, England, where the drug had been developed. They saw both animal trials and toxicological results. Both doctors had been seeking a drug with less harmful side effects and greater efficiency, and oxamniquine appeared to meet their requirements. However, they recognized that Brazil lacked both good volunteers that could be hospitalized for clinical testing and good clinical teams of pharmacologists.

The institute headed by Katz received funding from the National Research Council in Brazil, once the oxamniquine tests were programmed in 1970 for two and a half years; this provided for eighteen staff personnel, including four M.D.s.

Pfizer provided the drugs for testing, and the standards for the trials were developed among the professionals at Pfizer's lab in England and in the Brazilian institutes—a cooperation that was successful largely because the institutes had previous experience with the disease. The clinical testing started out with several different formulations of intramuscular doses, but all of them caused considerable pain in the area of application (buttocks). Some patients could not sit down or even lie down comfortably for a day or so. The IM dose is usually more effective, but an oral dose was developed and used because of greater comfort. Even so, some 10–20 percent of the people presently treated do not fully respond to the oral drug (at least egg production by the worms is not reduced significantly); therefore, they need a second or third dosage. If they are not cured then they can often be cured by an IM dose. The cost of conducting clinical trials after animal screening of the drug for schistosomiasis amounted to approximately $150,000—or $300 per person for some five hundred patients.

Preliminary Field Trials

With the development of the new oral form of oxamniquine, mass treatment to break the cycle of schistosomiasis appeared to be feasible. SUCAM decided that it would be necessary to demonstrate the efficacy of the drug in mass treatment in the field before presenting an overall control program to top government officials. It set up its own trial in the State of Paraná, where people from the Northeast had migrated with the disease, but where there was not yet an endemic infection (because snails were not generally infested). Pfizer provided the drugs for these trials. Of those treated, 96 percent were cured with no surprises as to risks. SUCAM concluded the drug was ready for mass use, so it moved next to a high-endemic area, where a large number of the people were continuously exposed to infections. Pfizer donated sufficient drugs to treat the entire population of Tourus, a village in the Northeast. In this trial, some side effects occurred in some patients, as expected from the clinical trial results. A few patients died during the program, but no more than the normal expectation without treatment in a population that size, so SUCAM did not consider these deaths drug-related. SUCAM recognized that there are risks in mass eradication programs but considered that its objectives were so important for the future of Brazil that it could not accept "excessively rigid" terms of reference of clinical researchers. The public health officer has a concept of "acceptable risk" for the community populace as a whole, while academic and clinical researchers emphasize the protection of each individual.

To try to get public health officers and academic researchers to work cooperatively together, SUCAM sponsored a national conference in Brazil in August 1977 on control of the disease and program implementation. This conference produced a three-volume report that included a number of conference papers and records of the field trials.[17] SUCAM officials concluded that the program was already contributing to the improvement of techniques of mass treatment, since they found that different dosages were not needed for different age groups, but rather that dosages should be graduated by the weight of the patient. The side effects of the drug were so insignificant that SUCAM stopped gathering statistics on them (though it watched for ill effects). Officials found that it was better not to ask the patients if they had any side effects because generally they answered positively, thinking that was what the interviewer wanted.

Following the success of the experimental programs in two regions, and with the approval of most of the experts at the conference, SUCAM was ready to seek approval for the large-scale program of control.

Approval Process and Control Design

A program of control had been proposed by SUCAM in 1972—four years before the present program was approved—but was passed over, partly because of the lack of priority assigned to schistosomiasis by the minister of health. A new minister in 1975 took up the program proposed by SUCAM with the president of Brazil, who agreed as to its importance. The program was considered by the Ministerial Social Development Council of the government, which is advisory to the president; it assessed the experimental results found from the two field trials and numerous statistical data on prevalence gathered by Pfizer.[18] An allocation of Cr$1.75 billion was approved by the president in July 1976.

The approval was based largely on the results of the field trials in Paraná and Tourus, which were documented with full statistical

[17] Ministerior da Saude, *Painel Programa*.
[18] The news media frequently discussed schistosomiasis and its spread across the country. Conselho de Desenvolvinmento Social, *Programa Especial de Controle de Esquistossomose no Brasil* (Brasília, 1976).

58

support, showing what was done, the results in terms of successful cure, follow-up tests, and all indications of side effects and their seriousness. This careful documentation convinced government officials that SUCAM could and would carry out a national program effectively and successfully. In addition, SUCAM had earlier achieved credibility through its successful vaccination of 80 million people against meningitis, despite the opposition of many professional experts, when an outbreak of the disease was threatened.

During the above approval process, some problems in the treatment of patients were used as arguments against the program: (1) In order to get cooperation from patients it is frequently necessary to treat symptoms rather than the disease itself; but in schistosomiasis, there are seldom any clear symptoms that the patient can recognize, and even when symptoms do exist (normally from serious cases), if they are relieved, the patient will feel that he is cured and will not continue treatment. (2) Reinfections do occur, through repeated exposure to worms in the water, with higher frequencies among children. (3) Danger for some people apparently arises from the worms becoming immobilized in the body, which may create respiratory and liver problems, though these appear to be rare. (4) Oxamniquine apparently kills the male but permits the female to live, though she cannot produce eggs alone; therefore, there is no continuing damage from new eggs, but the effects of her staying in the patient are not clinically known (her presence may help develop antibodies against new infections). (5) No one drug appears to be 100 percent effective against all cases even of *S. mansoni* (in clinical tests, oxamniquine was not found effective against *S. japonicum, S. haematobium*, or other strains of the disease). (6) Some persons simply cannot be treated because of pregnancy or some conditions of ill health.

Despite these problems, the Brazilian government concluded that the medical-sanitary and socioeconomic conditions prevalent in most rural areas would permit elimination or improvement of the disease to satisfactory levels. The pessimistic attitude toward schistosomiasis elimination changed to a positive attitude toward bringing the diseases "under control." "Under control" means the reduction of reinfections through the reduction of egg production by the worms in humans, which also reduces the effects of the disease. Individuals can live with the disease to some extent—that is, with worm infections maintained at a low level—without serious effects on the body. Although this may not be the most desirable result, it is at least achievable.

The program objective of control, rather than eradication, is supported by the results of research in a small government laboratory near the northeastern city of Natal, which had been examining wild animals to see if there is another schistosome cycle other than the one including humans. It found infestation in wild rats and mice and counted eggs in their feces, concluding that there is another cycle of infection. This means that it is impossible to eradicate the disease without killing all carrier snails (vectors) everywhere. Such an eradication is impossible to accomplish; therefore, the disease is likely to persist.

To break the human cycle, it is necessary to keep people out of the water. But SUCAM officials have had considerable difficulty in convincing some of the people of the need to do so, for this requires a change in cultural and work habits. In one instance, SUCAM technicians found a woman standing in a river full of infected snails, washing her clothes next to a low bridge. Asked if she did not understand the danger of the disease and the likelihood of becoming infected, she responded, "Yes, but where will I wash if not here?" The team reminded her of a nearby well from which she could draw good water and wash her clothes; she replied that the well was too far away, she would have to raise the water, and there was no convenient place to beat the clothes. Thus, not understanding the longer-term damage of the disease, she weighed short-term inconvenience more heavily.

Another obstacle to breaking the cycle of infestation is that it is also impossible to find all persons who are infected, so as to eliminate the chain in the human cycle. In a small city of 15,000 visited in the area of Natal, 1,000 were not treated because they were absent during the various medications. SUCAM technicians tried to pursue them by revisiting and tracing them; they cut the number of untreated to 600. At this point they abandoned the effort because the number of untreated was less than 4 percent of the population, which was SUCAM's cutoff figure.

Even though "control" was the objective, SUCAM considered that considerable benefit would accrue from the program in increased productivity of workers, in the educational capacity or attention of children, and in improvement in their sexual, physical, and mental development as a result of the elimination of the disease. Schistosomiasis produces general physical debility, reducing ability to concentrate. Public health officers found one eighteen-year-old boy with little intellectual development and no pubic hairs. SUCAM found some correlation between these effects and the number of eggs produced in the feces. A high egg-count is also correlated with lower than normal body weight and anemia, as well as susceptibility to other diseases; tuberculosis is more frequent and hepatitis is more serious among those with schistosomiasis.

Among the objectives of the program were, therefore: (1) reducing the numbers of people affected by the disease through the use of oral dosages of oxamniquine; (2) motivating communities to adopt preventive sanitation; (3) killing the snail hosts through molluscicides in the breeding areas; (4) avoiding new sources of the disease in water and irrigation projects; (5) avoiding migration of the disease; and (6) integrating the program with other government programs for the construction of adequate water supplies, sanitary sewers, laundries, and public bathrooms and for the improvement of home sanitation conditions.

SUCAM was not able to do a detailed cost-benefit analysis for the program; such an analysis is highly complex. University of Wisconsin researchers attempted to make such an analysis in Santa Lucia, but decided they could not reach firm conclusions.[19] Estimates made by a WHO official from studies in the Philippines counted the loss of productivity and the cost of health care for schistosomiasis at $6.5 million per year, or $25 per person—even larger than the recorded economic and social cost of malaria. In Egypt, the annual loss from the disease per person was estimated between $3.50 and $15.00, while the losses in Iraq and Japan amounted to $24 and $26 per person, respectively. The Egyptian study showed a 25 percent reduction in mistakes made by industrial workers and a 37.5 percent drop in absenteeism with a consequent increase of production by 12.5 percent—all as a result of the elimination of schistosomiasis in a given area. Official Brazilian estimates came to $20 per patient, which, when multiplied by the estimated 8–10 million infected persons, would suggest an annual loss of $160–200 million (or nearly Cr$3 billion).[20]

The original program proposal was estimated to cost Cr$100 per person (U.S. $8), totalling Cr$1.75 billion over four years. These funds were to support more than 3,000 people in the field, including lab technicians, those providing medication, control staff, supervisors, and auxiliary personnel. Some 13 million examinations were planned, with treatment of up to 12 million patients.

As indicated in the objectives, the program was to be coordi-

---

[19] R. E. Baldwin and B. A. Weisbrod, "Diseases and Labor Productivity," *Economic Development and Cultural Change*, vol. 22 (1974), pp. 414–35. A general study on health concluded that individuals in poor health were unemployed longer than those in good health. See P. L. Burgess and J. L. Kingston, "The Effect of Health on Duration of Employment," *Monthly Labor Review*, vol. 97, no. 4 (1974), pp. 53–54.
[20] Conselho de Desenvolvinmento Social, *Programa Especial*, p. 16.

nated with an environmental sanitation program undertaken by another agency within the Ministry of Health—Fundacão Serviços de Saude Publica (FSESP)—which helps build latrines, showers, and communal laundries, so as to keep these three activities out of community water sources. In addition to the above funding, Cr$800 million was projected from FSESP for help in sanitizing various areas of endemic disease. This raised the total to Cr$2.55 billion (at the rates of exchange then prevailing, U.S. $180 million) over the four-year period. The program was to cover over 2,000 municipalities and rural areas throughout the entire country, but concentrating initially on the Northeast and the areas between it and Brasília.

SUCAM proposed to begin treatment in late 1976 and to complete the basic program of control by 1979, but it actually did not begin until 1977, partly because of delayed delivery of 1,100 microscopes that were needed for the many field examinations in widely dispersed locations. Despite several delays, the program proceeded fairly rapidly once on its way because a cadre within SUCAM had been working on malaria, schistosomiasis, and other endemic diseases for some years and could train new personnel quickly. The existence of prior ongoing programs made it possible simply to meld the new campaign into the organization. Facilities for education and environmental sanitation and facilities for snail control were also in existence.

In the total program 4,000 personnel were projected as needed over the period 1976–1979 in all phases. It was necessary to train 1,400 new laboratory technicians, 470 new laboratory assistants, and 2,000 new field health care personnel. The latter are responsible for such tasks as the collection of feces for diagnosis (coproscopy) to determine who needs treatment, the collection of snails for examination of infestation (malacology), and the application of molluscicides in the infested snail-breeding areas, as well as treatment of other areas not yet infested.

The activities of all personnel were to be dovetailed with an intense campaign on sanitary education, employing audiovisual aids, to obtain the total cooperation of individuals and community and government units in the area. This work has continued after treatment was begun, so as to maintain high vigilance and attempt to change hygiene habits of the people. An FSESP project for basic sanitation facilities projected coverage of 233 municipalities and 1,366 localities (villages or smaller), directly helping 2.5 million people through the installation of 754 water supply systems, 875,000 household sanitary improvements, and 1,114 school sanitary improvements, plus construction of 741 public facilities for laundry, drinking water, and bathroom units.

Without this multipronged approach, reinfection would undo the medical treatment. SUCAM was given sole responsibility by the Ministry to coordinate all aspects of the program; it established a Special Program for Control of Schistosomiasis (PECE) to make certain that all activities and agencies appropriately phased and dovetailed. The difficulty of this coordination can be best understood if one recognizes that all of Brazil's watershed areas were included, save those in a few of the western and extreme southern states, comprising a territory nearly as large as the continental United States. The populace of some of these areas was 100 percent infected and would require extensive medication.

Analysis of the situation in the Northeast showed a majority of the population to be suffering from a number of diseases as a result of acute insufficiency of resources—material, financial, and technical. The people live in precarious health conditions stemming from poor sanitation, education, and housing. A large number would benefit from construction of water systems and any assistance in protecting their health against water-borne diseases. In the cities, water systems already existed and only needed to be improved and expanded. Although numerous city people are infected, they learn to stay out of the water themselves, so that the chain of infestation can be broken.

In the rural areas the highest priority is to raise the educational level of children to change their sanitation habits. At the request of SUCAM, Pfizer prepared a series of teaching aids, including contests, posters, and comic books to assist in getting student interest and compliance. The cooperation of municipal authorities and the people is necessary in improving sanitation through constructing laundries, bathing facilities, water supplies, and sewers. Some of the costs of this construction can be borne by the communities themselves, either with municipal funds or with work contributed directly by the people in the area.

Instruction on vigilance began with the community-centered involvement in the schools, but the word spread quickly to other sectors in society through formal and informal groups. In cities, business, professional, and youth groups are effective; in rural areas, the schools are places for association. Health officers are trained to describe how to recognize the symptoms and effects of the disease, what is needed in terms of sanitary facilities, and how the community can do its part. A number of materials and manuals were developed to train teachers, who could then instruct the students—using charts, portfolios, films, and albums to collect and display information. Community Health Patrols were organized to sensitize teachers to the health needs of the community, to train teachers in sanitary education, to train people no longer in schools to form their own neighborhood health patrols, and to assess the progress of the various community works.

Surveillance must continue, even after the medication campaign in the Northeast is completed. Though personnel in that area can then be reduced by roughly two-thirds and shifted to other areas, maintenance personnel must remain because complete control will still not have been achieved.

Despite this planning, PECE underestimated the problems of control. They occur in both the snail and the human phases of the cycle. The snail, which is the host to the parasite, is very smart in its environment. It is one of the oldest forms of life on earth and has been able to adjust to a great deal of change. It carries its own house in the shell and procreates without a mate, if necessary. The parasite (schistosome) is a hearty species, known to be at least five thousand years old. The attack should be on it rather than on the snail, which is an unwilling host in the cycle. The ease of killing parasites or snails was underestimated.

In order to break the chain, teams must work on human sanitation (customs of defecation) and stop the human phase of the gestation of eggs in the human host. But it is extremely difficult to change the human habits of centuries of using any available open water for defecation, baths, and laundry. Even when sanitation officials have been able to persuade people in a community not to defecate in the water, the people have continued to wash themselves after defecation, leaving eggs in the water and completing the cycle.

Program Implementation

In the field the five parts of the program—snail counting (malacology), countering of infected persons (coproscopy), medication, snail eradication, and sanitation—were combined differently according to the following guidelines:

- in special project areas, coproscopical survey of the entire population, treatment of all cases plus follow-up to assure cure control, and malacological survey and application of molluscicides in snail-breeding areas

- in areas where snails are not yet infected, survey of prevalence among students, treatment of those testing positive and their families, checks to assure cure control, and malacological survey and application of molluscicides in breeding areas

- in areas with small transmission, coproscopy of students only, treatment of the entire population where infection is above 50 percent (because in a single sampling numerous "false negatives" are found which would imply much greater infection), cure control by post-treatment evaluation through sampling of students, treatment of those tested positive and later cure control where the infection rate is below 50 percent, and malacological survey and control in both areas

- in all areas, development or improvement of sanitation facilities, and educational activities to alert the communities and to motivate them to change their sanitation habits.

The first step in implementation was the taking of samples of feces to determine the incidence of the disease and therefore the level of treatment to be given (if any). This was done by visits of technical teams to schools or selected houses in a village. They explained the program and left containers for the individual feces, to be labeled appropriately, collected later, and sent to one of the laboratories for egg count (coproscopic examination).

Once it was determined that the disease existed in an area, the second stage (malacology) was begun, to determine the location and extent of snail transmission. Since any body of water is likely to be used by the populace and could be a source of infection, every lake, stream, pond, or water source was located and mapped by a technical team. The mapping was rough and by hand, but precise enough for a molluscicide team to determine where the water was and its relative size. The team circled the entire body of water or traversed the stream or river and took samples from it along the bank and out to two or three meters at locations roughly 50 meters apart. A strainer on a long handle was dipped into the water and the soft bottom and through weeds and grasses in the water to pick up any snails. This dipping was done five times to the left of the spot and five times to the right, so as to gain adequate coverage. If any snails were found, they were taken back in sealed bags, marked with the location. The spot where the snails were taken is marked precisely at the water's edge and on the map. One of the teams observed during the research visit required a full day to examine three small ponds near the ocean at São Bento do Norte.

In the microscopic examination, several snails from a single location were placed on a small glass plate, with another similar plate placed on top. The snails were then crushed by hand between the two plates permitting internal examination by microscope. If they were found to be infested, their source was marked for later application of molluscicides. Whether or not infestation was found, records were kept by the lab of the number of snails brought in from each location and the number of those examined (usually 100 percent), with the degree of infestation noted.

The results of the snail survey were also used to determine the area for coproscopic sampling. São Bento do Norte is at the edge of the infected areas in that part of the Northeast, but SUCAM was not sure how far westward the infected area extended. The only activity in that area at the time of the visit was the snail survey, to determine the extent of infestation and potential infection of humans. Once these results were in, the coproscopic teams would come in, if needed, followed by the sanitation and treatment teams. In this region, much of the water was stagnant rainwater caught in drainage areas. Running water or water which has a high saline content because of proximity to the ocean is much less likely to have snails than is stagnant fresh water. Every body of water in the area, even if not used by the population, was examined in order to get a fix on possible snail transmission. If no snails were found, no further steps were taken, but records were retained for future reference.

The research visit included the opportunity to observe the medication program. One village with SUCAM officials was about a half-hour drive through rural areas outside of Natal; another was two-and-a-half hours by jeep into the littoral of Northeast Brazil. In each case, SUCAM teams numbered the houses to provide a continuous census of the village. House 128, for example, was made of stucco over woven branches (mud wattle) for the walls, with a roof of woven sticks. The house was about fifteen feet by fifteen feet, with three rooms and a dirt floor. The father was thirty-three years old, and the mother appeared to be older, with seven children aged two to twelve. One of the children had a fever and was given no medication; two were too small to receive capsules and received the medication in syrup; three were given pills which they took quite readily; and a seventh was at school, where he obtained medication from another SUCAM team. The parents themselves were not given medication because the incidence of schistosomiasis in the area was less than 20 percent. After the medication was given, a mimeographed sheet was pasted to the back of the door recording the visit and the medication given. Already in place were two other pieces of paper showing the results of the census and the earlier coproscopy. Not all houses had all three sheets, since the feces examination was done on a sampling basis.

After treating patients in houses 128 and 129, the medication team looked for 130, which was supposed to be across the dirt street. They could not find it and thought that someone might have erased a number or played a trick, but neighbors finally told them that the house had been washed away by the rains and the people were in another location. This location was not on their map, but they had to pursue the people to their new living quarters.

The medication phase was conducted by teams of two public health officers dressed in uniforms with the SUCAM name and military style caps—one officer carrying the weight scales for determining dosage and another the medication and records. Three different medication teams were operating in the village at the time. The teams appeared to be paired by age and probably by experience as well. One was composed of two fairly young men (between twenty-five and thirty), the second of men around forty-five, and the third of men who appeared to be fifty-five to sixty.

Each inspector for a given area had five teams of two technicians each, recruited from the general area in which they worked, so that they not only knew the people but had a direct interest in the program's success. The SUCAM official guessed that the technicians were paid between Cr$25,000–30,000, or a maximum of $2,000 per year (at July 1977 exchange rates); the technicians on these teams would have probably had no more than five years of school and inspectors would have reached seventh to ninth grades. In addition to the two technicians, a young woman was accompanying one team to help explain to the families, if necessary, the desirability of taking the medication. The courtesy, thoughtfulness, and helpfulness of the teams was remarkable.

It took a team a full day to treat the inhabitants of fifteen houses, despite the fact that the houses were usually close together. If the parents were away, as they often were, the team had to return when they were there. The children in the neighborhood often became excited with the activity and followed from house-to-house, so that by the end of the day a team's entourage reached between twenty and thirty onlookers. In one house, at least twelve people were packed in an eight-by-ten-foot room, watching the proceedings, while others were hanging through the windows. These kibitzers were useful because they reinforced the willingness of others to cooperate; the children especially took their medicine more readily in the presence of their friends. The eagerness of the very young children to take the medicine resulted partly from the fact that the syrup was sweet and they were given the plastic spoon, which they continued to lick like a sucker.

The care with which the technical team covered the village was striking. One technician had made a hand-drawn map of the area, and each house was placed on the map in sequence with its number. Once the occupants of a house were treated, the fact was noted on the map, leaving those not reached unmarked. All houses were visited according to their numbers, the teams zigzagging across the street, rather than proceeding down one side at a time. (In one village, the team had to cross and recross a large ditch down the middle of the dirt road being dug for sewer drainage by local workers under the direction of FSESP.)

A written record was kept of all names of individuals at each house, their age, weight, sex, and dosage given, along with any observations on each—such as contraindications, inability to give the medicine because of illness, or "at school." The inspectors and technicians were trained to recognize such contraindications as fever, disease, heart attack, and malaria, as well as certain side effects. They were given two-month courses, with some description of and exposure to the nature and the development of schistosomiasis.

The area under each inspector was divided into territories where teams were assigned. A linear path marked on a map showed where each team was to follow in daily work, beginning at one end of the territory and ending at the other. The territories were elongated to eliminate doubling back to cover a village. Each area was designed to be covered in a set number of days. Since a census had already been taken, the technicians were provided with the appropriate number of dosages and instruction as to who was to be treated. Once one village was covered, the team moved on to the next until all villages in the region were covered.

Observations of the program in operation made it evident that one of its most important aspects was the extensive and precise record-keeping at all stages. Only through this could SUCAM be certain that the program was carried out as intended. To fill out and maintain these records required a dedication to detail which was surprising, at least to this observer, in view of the lack of familiarity with such procedures, the relative independence of the teams, and their distance from authority. It could only have been done through careful instruction and a personal commitment by technicians to the community and its continuing health.

5

The Future

The problems facing those who seek to eradicate or reduce the presence of the six tropical diseases are numerous and complex, and they arise from quite varied sources—medical, political, economic, and bureaucratic. In order to assess the future roles of the pharmaceutical companies in controlling the six diseases, we need to distinguish the medical aspects, the political, and the economic. Among medical research priorities, the six special diseases are not high, since other diseases are larger incapacitators or killers and in more countries. The six have proven intractable, but a shift in research emphasis will have to come as a response to pressures other than medical. Political pressure has arisen, giving the six a special priority which can elicit emotional responses for extended assistance. From the economic standpoint, emphasis on these six depends, as shown in the foregoing study, on the willingness of governments to reallocate budgets and resources so as to generate delivery systems and markets that will elicit company resources. Future dialogues among companies, governments, and international organizations should keep all three aspects in mind and attempt to bring them closer together so that priorities are reinforcing.

In meeting the problems of these tropical diseases, governments and companies would need to engage in several stages of activity, some in sequence and some simultaneously. The complexities and variations of these stages reflect the weaving together of medical, political, economic, and administrative elements at the industry, national, and international levels—each institution having a different role to play. The sequence of stages is as follows:

1. Identification of medical need is the first stage. It can be done by one or more of several entities—individual doctors, public health officials, health ministries, company personnel (marketing or re-

search), private international health groups, intergovernmental health institutions, and so on. Companies can play an important role here, but theirs is not determinant, for a need may exist that companies do not recognize. Even if they *do* recognize a need, they will not necessarily respond by action at the second stage. The need must be translated into a demand which will bear the costs of drug development and delivery. Companies differ even in their assessment as to adequate demand: some may respond positively to certain market signals, while others do not.

2. Drug development follows in response to the specification of the need to be met. The company role is dominant here (or the role may be assumed by an independent or government laboratory) in that a commitment of R & D resources must be made—in competition with other needs or opportunities. The decision is constrained—as illustrated earlier—by company orientations, resources, specialization, capabilities, and preferences of scientists. Development begins with discovery of a compound or agent that is effective against the disease. Proper formulations, dosages, and toxicity limits must then be determined. Success in these areas is followed by clinical trials for testing safety and efficacy in humans. The location of these tests is often mandated by governments; some do not accept results found in another country.

3. Commercialization follows if clinical success is achieved, and regulatory bodies approve, along with a scale-up of the production process to commercial volumes. Having identified a market, the company seeks to determine the size of the market, given the characteristics of the drug developed and its costs. That is, the company seeks to place the drug in its market niche. If possible, the drug will have been patented so that it can obtain a price which will repay the extensive costs of development. Finally, the drug must be distributed. All of these activities are largely the responsibility of the pharmaceutical companies, save the regulatory approvals of the results of the clinical trials. In case of tropical diseases, three problems are injected in this process: the companies do not always have facilities *in situ* for clinical trials; the markets are not known or developed; and distribution requires a large delivery system involving governments. Consequently, further steps are necessary—in which the companies are not dominant.

4. Where mass distribution is needed, field trials are also required. The drug must be taken into the country where the disease exists and be applied under existing environmental and social conditions. The purpose of these tests is to determine the feasibility of a large-scale eradication program; they need to determine the probability of success so as to justify budget allocation.

70

These trials are seldom the responsibility of the companies, in part because they are more expensive than the companies will undertake on their own and in part because the governments want the assessment of their own scientists. Field trials will, therefore, require cooperation between the companies and national governments; where the latter do not have adequate resources or appropriate capabilities, assistance by WHO would be in order.

5. Adoption of special programs of eradication by national governments is the next stage, after successful field trials. Approval of such programs will generally occur only after consideration of costs and benefits to the country. This step is probably the most critical of all, since without it nothing further will be done. The responsibility for this step is almost wholly with national governments, though the World Bank and the UN Development Program (UNDP) can provide funding for some of the studies necessary or even perform the cost-benefit studies themselves; companies would not be involved in view of potential conflict of interest.

6. An effective delivery system is required in order to implement a disease control or eradication program. This will include the infrastructure of public health services, a training program for public health officers, governmental administrators, teachers, and supporting personnel, and an appreciation of local cultures so that the techniques adopted or prescribed are successfully implemented. Like the adoption stage discussed above, this stage is almost wholly the responsibility of the national government, and it represents a considerable obstacle where public health services do not already exist. Even where they do exist, there will be additional costs for training and direct implementation, plus the necessary drugs, and these can be extensive, as is seen in the Brazilian program on schistosomiasis. However, pharmaceutical companies can and do assist in the training of technicians in proper medication or lab procedure.

7. A nonmedication phase of vector control is necessary in most of the tropical diseases so as to prevent reinfection by breaking the cycle of infestation at the insect or carrier junction. This requires application of different types of chemicals (pesticides or molluscicides) and efforts to improve the environment so as to reduce the number and size of locations where the vectors can survive (ideally, reduced to zero). The responsibility for this stage is largely that of national governments; however, assistance can be obtained from WHO and possibly from UNDP, and sometimes from the companies supplying necessary chemical agents. In most instances, this stage is a cooperative effort.

8. Environmental conditions will have to be changed in order to improve general health and reduce the likelihood of infestation

from tropical diseases, since they are environment-related. Improvement in general sanitation (water use, fly control, bathing, for example) will be required. Although this stage is the responsibility of the community and the national government, some assistance can be obtained from WHO and other international agencies.

9. Education will be required in several directions: in the proper use of the drug and the reasons for taking it; in vector control and the significance of continued attention to this control; and in the need for improvements in sanitation and cultural changes and the methods of accomplishing them. This is also the responsibility of the national government or the local community, but pharmaceutical companies can and have assisted in the preparation of educational materials and training of teachers.

10. Local facilities for training and research and development will be required to assist developing countries in making appropriate judgments on methods of control in eradicating the tropical diseases and on the desirability of doing so. These facilities should also lead to improvements in techniques of disease control as experiments are conducted in local environments. These local capabilities are important also in program determination—as is seen in the reliance on local scientists for government approval of the Brazilian schistosomiasis program. These capabilities will eventually support the move toward local production of pharmaceuticals, on which many countries insist.

This summary of the stages required to mount campaigns against the six tropical diseases shows that pharmaceutical companies have only a limited role to play in the "total program." This role is primarily in drug development, but success in this area is difficult to achieve, given the necessary characteristics of drugs and vaccines for control or eradication campaigns. The drugs must be produced at a cost that can be borne by the developing countries infested with these diseases; their distribution and use must require minimal skills and limited specialized supervision; and their distribution must be feasible through the public health services of LDCs. These conditions place some very serious constraints on the companies in drug development, which may mean that R & D resources will be turned toward other objectives—unless market or other incentives arise. To close the gap between needs and resources and between program criteria of government and companies, it will probably be necessary to develop some new cooperative or institutional arrangements.

During the interviews, several company officials stressed the necessity to look for new approaches to offset the normal pull of more attractive commercial areas. Continuous support for R & D effort on tropical diseases requires an interest in both the R & D (the curiosity to see whether compounds can be developed and adapted to wide usage) and in the marketing departments of a company and their active involvement, despite the fact that there might not be a large financial return. Such an orientation can be stimulated by governments of the advanced countries either through tax incentives (R & D deductions) or application of aid funds for basic research in chemotherapy or immunology and for funding delivery systems abroad. National and international aid agencies could support development of particular drugs by giving to companies with appropriate expertise contracts that include the costs of toxicology and preclinical tests.

Only with this type of cooperation between governments and companies can industry facilities be used most effectively. Companies are willing to bear their portion of the costs in development of chemotherapeutic agents, plus clinical testing and production. Such costs were estimated by one company to require nearly $10 million per year, with a minimum of 100 scientific and technical personnel in one laboratory working on the two diseases of malaria and schistosomiasis. But the government would have to complement the effort by assuming responsibility for field trials and by providing a continuing market through mass treatment programs.

In order to meld the phases of company initiatives, host government delivery systems, and funding, one company official suggested that WHO should assign two developing countries to each major pharmaceutical company, with the company undertaking to eradicate or control, say, two diseases (for example, TB and leprosy). The funds for each project would be provided from the local government, WHO, and the World Bank or regional development banks. Companies should then accept lower returns from such a project or adopt "project accounting," using the profits from any given project for further development of research in tropical disease areas—that is, keeping the returns in the same project field.

Another company suggested a similarly dispersed "total program," which would include the following: (1) drug development in selected centers, under the direction of a single company; (2) basic research by universities under WHO coordination; (3) protocols designed by industry for clinical testing; (4) clinical work by WHO or local hospitals or laboratories; (5) cooperative research among a very few (probably no more than five) companies (depending on the interest of the various companies, cooperation can be guided effectively if there is a careful spelling out of responsibilities and rights by each part); (6) coordinated intergovernmental approval of drugs for mass application, so as to reduce duplication of clinical tests and animal screening; (7) national and international funding; and (8) development of centers of disease control in such cities as Bombay and Nairobi, with much later development of R & D capabilities in local laboratories.

These proposals are far reaching, but they are grounded in an understanding of the need for a "total program" approach for control of the six diseases. The companies can play only a limited role, given the competing claims on their resources and the need for governmental action in most of the program phases. But these proposals can never succeed unless the traditional adversarial positions of business and government are replaced by a cooperative attitude in jointly attacking the serious problems affecting the productivity and growth of many developing countries.

Date Due

MAY 09 '90			
MAY 31 '93	04 30 07		

RC 961.5 .B43   303382

BEHRMAN, JACK N.

TROPICAL DISEASES